Chemical-Induced Seizures: Mechanisms, Consequences and Treatment

Editor

Feng Ru Tang, MD, Ph.D

Temasek Laboratories,
National University of Singapore,
5A, Engineering Drive 1,
Singapore 117411
E-mail: tangfr@gmail.com

Co-Editor

Weng Keong Loke, Ph.D

Defence Medical and Environmental Research Institute,
DSO National Laboratories,
11 Stockport Road,
Singapore 117605
E-mail: lwengkeo@dso.org.sg

CONTENTS

FOREWORD

In recent history, chemical warfare nerve agents have been used as a weapon in the battlefield as well as an instrument to spread panic by terrorists on innocent public. Unfortunately, because of limited scientific interest, there are not many laboratories engaged in chemical defence research in the world to help mitigate the threats. Hence, several gaps still exist in understanding of the toxic effects of such agents in the victims for the immediate and longer term. For example, we do not have a thorough understanding on the pathophysiological and behavioural changes after nerve agent poisoning to help us explain the psychological, mental effects and neurological impairment reported in victims with chronic signs and systems. This situation is not helped by the lack of experience and scarcity of clinical cases in daily clinical practice; doctors hardly ever see patients whose conditions have any similarity to casualties of nerve agent intoxication.

Drs Feng Ru Tang and Weng Keong Loke from Singapore are to be commended for this initiative to edit and organize an E-book, *"Chemical-induced seizures: mechanisms, consequences and treatment"*. It represents a collection of the latest scientific understanding in this topic of nerve agents and their deleterious impact from the relatively limited number of world renowned specialists in this field. Furthermore each article list several relevant references thus collating into this E-book the relevant information from publications and articles, which are currently spread over a wide range of journals and books. Both Dr Tang and Dr Loke have been researching in epilepsy and in the medical effects of chemical warfare agents for many years. I am confident that this book will not only benefit scientists, and doctor but also policy and emergency planners for national emergencies and security.

Professor Lionel Lee
Defence Medical and Environmental Research Institute,
DSO National Laboratories,
Singapore.

PREFACE

At the turn of the 20th century, following the Tokyo Sarin Subway Attack, the threat of chemical warfare agents has migrated from the battlefield to become a major concern for homeland security in the 21st century. While current fielded antidotes are able to mitigate acute high mortality arising from exposure to nerve agents, achieving effective neuroprotection in subjects with nerve agent induced prolonged seizures or status epilepticus is currently lacking. To overcome this challenge, establishing an improved understanding on the mechanism linking seizure onset during chemical (including nerve agents) poisoning to the subsequent cascade of biochemical, neurotoxicological, pathophysiological, genomic and behavioral changes post exposure is vital. Due to ethical, safety and chemical surety related issues, looking for surrogate chemicals also become important for chemical defense research. In this book, internationally well-known clinicians and basic research scientists with expertise on chemical-induced seizures will update readers on the relevant areas. In Chapter 1, Lee and Kales, review the basic principles of seizure generation, relevant microscopic neuroanatomy, neuroelectrophysiology, neurotoxicology and molecular genetics along with specific examples of chemicals known to elicit seizures. In Chapters 2 and 3, Feiner et al. and Dolkart et al. present nerve agent-induced neurological symptoms, diagnosis of nerve agent intoxication, pre-hospital assistance and intra-hospital management of seizures. In Chapter 4, Joosen et al. discuss about specific neuroanatomical routes for soman-induced seizure generation and spreading, neurotoxicology profiles and effects on neurogenesis and cognition. Loke and Ho summarize their research findings in Chapter 5 and suggest that manipulating central α_2-adrenergic and cholinergic receptors may produce neuroprotective effects in nerve agent poisoned animals with established status epilepticus. In Chapters 6, 7, 8, seizure models induced by other chemicals are reviewed by Aker *et al.*, Tang *et al.*, Tang and Loke respectively. Tang and Loke systemically compare the mechanisms of seizure generation, the subsequent neuropathological, genomic, and neurobehavioral changes between pilocarpine- and nerve agent-induced seizure models, and suggest that pilocarpine model may be a surrogate model for nerve agent-induced seizures. Doctors (civil and military), paramedics and medical students will find this book informative and timely for the current battle against asymmetric terrorist conflicts.

Dr. Feng Ru Tang
Temasek Laboratories,
Singapore

Dr. Weng Keong Loke
Defence Medical and Environmental Research Institute,
Singapore

LIST OF CONTRIBUTORS

Rezzan Gülhan Aker

Department of Pharmacology and Clinical Pharmacology, Marmara University School of Medicine, Istanbul, Turkey

Sergei Bankoul

Swiss Armed Forces, Office of the Surgeon in Chief, Ittigen, 3063 Switzerland, and Swiss Armed Forces, NBC Centre of Competence, Spiez, 3700, Switzerland

Christophe Baumberger

Swiss Armed Forces, NBC Centre of Competence, Spiez, 3700, Switzerland

Ron Ben-Abraham

Post Anesthesia Care Unit and Animal Research Laboratory, Tel Aviv Sourasky Medical Center, and the Sackler Faculty of Medicine, Tel Aviv University, Tel Aviv, Israel

Pierre-Nicolas Carron

Emergency Service, University Hospital (CHUV), Lausanne, 1011 Switzerland

Oleg Dolkart

Post Anesthesia Care Unit and Animal Research Laboratory, Tel Aviv Sourasky Medical Center, and the Sackler Faculty of Medicine, Tel Aviv University, Tel Aviv, Israel

Adam-Scott Feiner

Emergency Service, University Hospital (CHUV), Lausanne, 1011 Switzerland, Switzerland

Lai Kwan Ho

Defence Medical and Environmental Research Institute, DSO National Laboratories, 11 Stockport Road, Singapore 117605

Stefanos N. Kales

Harvard Medical School & Harvard School of Public Health, Medical Director, Employee & Industrial Medicine, Cambridge Health Alliance, 1493 Cambridge Street, Macht Bldg, The Cambridge Hospital Room 427, Cambridge, MA 02139, United States

Koichi Kato

Department of Neurosurgery, Tokyo Rosai Hospital
Address correspondence to: Dr. Koichi Kato, 4-13-21 Omoriminami, Ota-ku, Tokyo, 143-0013, Japan

Demet Kinay

I. Neurology Clinic, Bakirköy Research Hospital for Neurology, Neurosurgery and Psychiatry, Istanbul, Turkey

Marloes J.A. Joosen

TNO Defence, Security and Safety, Department of Chemical Toxicology, Lange Kleiweg 137, 2288GJ, Rijswijk, The Netherlands

Ernest C. Lee

Harvard School of Public Health, Senior Medical Officer, Occupational Health Detachment, Marine Corps Logistics Base Barstow, Bldg 149 James L Day St, Barstow, CA 92311, United States

Weng Keong Loke

Defence Medical and Environmental Research Institute, DSO National Laboratories, 11 Stockport Road, Singapore 117605

Filiz Yilmaz Onat

Department of Pharmacology and Clinical Pharmacology, Marmara University School of Medicine, Istanbul, Turkey

August B. Smit

Center for Neurogenomics and Cognitive Research, Free University, De Boelelaan 1085, 1081HV, Amsterdam, The Netherlands

Andreas Stettbacher

Swiss Armed Forces, Office of the Surgeon in Chief, Ittigen, 3063 Switzerland, Switzerland

Feng Ru Tang

Temasek Laboratories, National University of Singapore, 5A, Engineering Drive 1, Singapore 117411
Department of Anatomy, Yong Loo Lin School of Medicine, Block MD 10, National University of Singapore, 4 Medical Drive, Singapore 117597

Marcel J. van der Schans

TNO Defence, Security and Safety, Department of Chemical Toxicology, Lange Kleiweg 137, 2288GJ, Rijswijk, The Netherlands

Herman P.M. van Helden

TNO Defence, Security and Safety, Department of Chemical Toxicology, Lange Kleiweg 137, 2288GJ, Rijswijk, The Netherlands

Avi A Weinbroum

Post Anesthesia Care Unit and Animal Research Laboratory, Tel Aviv Sourasky Medical Center, and the Sackler Faculty of Medicine, Tel Aviv University, Tel Aviv, Israel

Bertrand Yersin

Emergency Service, University Hospital (CHUV), Lausanne, 1011 Switzerland

Genetic, Molecular, Neuroanatomic, and Electrophysiologic Mechanisms of Chemically Induced Seizures

Ernest C. Lee and Stefanos N. Kales[*]

Harvard Medical School & Harvard School of Public Health, Medical Director, Employee & Industrial Medicine, Cambridge Health Alliance, 1493 Cambridge Street, Macht Bldg, The Cambridge Hospital Room 427, Cambridge, MA 02139, United States

Abstract: Traditionally, chemically-induced seizures have received little detailed emphasis in general neurology literature. The few articles that describe correlations between seizures and chemical exposure(s) usually focus on clinical effects rather than underlying pathophysiological mechanisms. Conclusions of studies from various biological disciplines are discussed in order to convey a global understanding of chemically-induced seizure mechanisms. Theoretical mechanisms underlying the progression from a seizure occurring only with external induction to a seizure occurring spontaneously (epilepsy) are also discussed. A generally accepted model of epileptogensis is that of kindling, in which the clinical manifestations of seizures increase as seizures are repeatedly induced. Recent studies are beginning to reveal just how this kindling phenomenon might occur through permanent genetic and microneuroanatomic alterations induced by aberrant excessive electrical impulse activity, *via* direct physiologic injury, or through unintended adverse consequences of repair mechanisms. Large-scale genomic studies are beginning to reveal that many genes likely contribute to seizure induction and the loss of synaptic plasticity observed in epilepsy. Examples of mechanisms underlying specific chemically-induced seizures are discussed including those caused by cyanide, carbon monoxide, and chemical nerve agents. Further research and understanding of fundamental seizure mechanisms will likely lead to the discovery of novel and more effective methods by which to treat and ultimately prevent seizure or epilepsy development. To this end, a review of the basic principles of relevant microscopic neuroanatomy, neuroelectrophysiology, neurotoxicology, and molecular genetics, is presented along with specific examples of chemicals known to elicit seizures.

INTRODUCTION

General Principles of Seizures and Epileptogenesis

Traditionally, chemically-induced seizures have received little detailed emphasis in general neurology literature. The few articles that do describe correlations between seizures and chemical exposure(s) usually only describe clinical effects, but do not describe or speculate on the underlying pathophysiological mechanisms. Research increasingly indicates that various chemicals can adversely affect neuron synaptic transmission through a myriad of pathways. Neuron firing and transmission are complex multi-step, sequential processes. Hence there are many vulnerable anatomic areas and cellular processes that chemicals can affect in order to elicit seizure activity. Thus, improved understanding of the pathophysiological mechanisms of chemically induced seizures will not only allow development of methods to prevent seizures, but can potentially lead to development of medications to treat seizures.

There is a fine balance in the brain between factors that initiate electrical activity and factors that restrict it. Various systems limit the spread of electrical activity. In general, seizure activity occurs when a group of neurons in the cerebral cortex activate simultaneously emitting excessive bursts of electrical energy [1]. While the etiology of seizure activity can be determined in some cases, in the vast majority of cases the cause is unknown.

When seizures or the transient symptoms of excessive neuronal activity recur without provocation, this is known as epilepsy [2]. There are several theories as to why epilepsy might develop after recurrent seizure activity. A generally accepted model is that of kindling, in which the clinical manifestations of seizures increase as seizures are repeatedly induced. At a certain point, seizures begin to recur spontaneously even in the absence of external induction [3]. Recent studies are beginning to reveal just how this kindling phenomenon might occur through permanent genetic and

*Address correspondence to Dr. Stefanos N Kales: Associate Professor, Harvard Medical School & Harvard School of Public Health, Medical Director, Employee & Industrial Medicine, Cambridge Health Alliance, 1493 Cambridge Street, Macht Bldg, The Cambridge Hospital Room 427, Cambridge, MA 02139, United States; Tel: 617.665.1580; E-mail: skales@hsph.harvard.edu

Feng Ru Tang and Weng Keong Loke (Eds)

microneuroanatomic alterations induced by aberrant excessive electrical impulse activity, via direct physiologic injury, or through adverse consequences which can occasionally be the product of repair mechanisms [3-5].

MICROSCOPIC NEUROANATOMY AND ELECTROPHYSIOLOGY

A review of the basic principles of relevant microscopic neuroanatomy, neuroelectro-physiology, neurotoxicology, molecular genetics, is essential in order to understand and appreciate the various mechanisms by which chemicals can induce seizure activity.

The basic unit of the nervous system is the neuron, which is capable of conducting action potentials that are actual measurable electrical currents. The central part of the neuron is known as the soma, containing the nucleus, where most cellular protein synthesis occurs. Projecting from the body are numerous short processes known as dendrites, which are cellular extensions with many branches. These receive impulses from other neurons. A single long process known as the axon conducts nerve impulse away from the cell body and out to other neurons, muscles, and glands. Oftentimes an axon will undergo extensive branching, enabling communication with many target cells. The part of the axon emerging from the soma is called the axon hillock. It has the greatest density of voltage-dependent sodium channels thus making it the most easily excited part of the neuron and the spike initiation zone for the axon. While the axon is generally involved in information outflow, this region can also receive input from other neurons.

The site of contact between the axon and dendrite is known as the synapse. Electrical impulses signal neurons to release chemical mediators known as neurotransmitters across the synapse. Within a neuron, microtubules are used to transport neurotransmitters from their site of production in the cell body to the end of axons for release. Microtubules are small tubes formed by filamentous strands. Each filament strand is composed of a chain of protein called tubulin. Microtubules, microfilaments, and neurofilaments compose the cytoskeletal elements of a neuron. The dynamic behavior of neuronal filament proteins is under the control of protein kinases and phosphatases, which are enzymes that regulate the molecular activity at the ends of these structural proteins [7].

If a CNS nerve fiber is traumatically cut at the axon level, the part of the axon separated from the neuron's soma degenerates in a process known as anterograde or Wallerian degeneration. Anterograde degeneration begins within 24 hours after the axon is severed. The distal axonal skeleton disintegrates and the axonal membrane breaks apart. This is followed by degradation of the myelin sheath by microglia [8]. The rate of myelin clearance is very slow in the CNS and could play factor in the limited regeneration capabilities of the CNS. Glial cells also form scar tissue around the area of injury.

There are several classes of neurons. An important class with respect to seizures is the pyramidal neuron found in areas of the brain including the cerebral cortex, the hippocampus, and in the amygdala. Pyramidal neurons are the primary excitation units of the mammalian prefrontal cortex and the corticospinal tract [9]. Pyramidal neurons, like other neurons, have numerous voltage-gated ion channels. In pyramidal cells, there is an abundance of Na+, Ca2+, and K+ channels in the dendrites, and some channels in the soma. Ion channels within pyramidal cell dendrites have different properties from the same ion channel type within the pyramidal cell soma. Voltage-gated Ca2+ channels in pyramidal cell dendrites are activated by subthreshold excitatory postsynaptic potentials (EPSPs) and by back-propagating action potentials. The extent of back-propagation of impulses within pyramidal dendrites depends upon the K+ channels. K+ channels in pyramidal cell dendrites provide a mechanism for controlling the amplitude of action potentials [10].

The ability of pyramidal neurons to integrate information depends on the number and distribution of the synaptic inputs they receive. A single pyramidal cell receives about 30,000 excitatory inputs also known as EPSPs and 1700 inhibitory inputs otherwise known as inhibitory postsynaptic potentials (IPSPs). IPSP inputs terminate on dendritic shafts, the soma, and even the axon. EPSP inputs terminate exclusively on the dendritic spines. In general, pyramidal neurons use glutamate as their excitatory neurotransmitter, and GABA as their inhibitory neurotransmitter [11].

In addition to neurons, the nervous tissue also contains glial cells, which are support cells. There is approximately one glia for every neuron in the human brain [12]. Traditionally glia were not believed to play a role in neurotransmitter release; however, recent data indicate that glia participate in synaptic transmission, help regulate the clearance of neurotransmitters from the synaptic cleft, modulate presynaptic function by releasing factors such as

ATP, and even release neurotransmitters themselves [13]. Glial cells are classified into several types, the most relevant of which will be discussed here. The first type is microglia named because of their small size relative to macroglial cells. Microglial cells are specialized macrophages capable of phagocytosis acting as scavengers that multiply when neural tissue is damaged.

The most abundant type of macroglial cells are the astrocytes. Astrocytes anchor neurons to their blood supply, regulate the external chemical environment by removing excess ions, and recycle neurotransmitters. They are presumed to be the main component of the blood-brain barrier. Astrocytes contribute to the origins of epileptogenesis [14].

The outermost layer of the mammalian cerebrum is known as the cerebral cortex and is made up of six horizontal layers. Each layer has a different composition in terms of neurons and connectivity. Characteristic connections exist between different cortical layers and neuronal types, which span the entire thickness of the cortex. These cortical microcircuits are grouped into cortical columns and minicolumns, the latter of which have been proposed to be the basic functional units of cortex. White matter below the cortex is formed predominantly by myelinated axons interconnecting neurons in different regions of the cerebral cortex with each other and neurons in other parts of the central nervous system. The six classically recognized layers of the cortex include:

I.   Outer molecular layer: which contains sparse neurons and glial cells.

II. Outer granular layer: which contains small pyramidal and stellate neurons.

III. External pyramidal layer: contains moderate sized pyramidal neurons as well as non-pyramidal neurons with vertically-oriented intracortical axons.

IV. Internal granular layer: densely packed stellate neurons and pyramidal neurons.

V.   Ganglionic or internal pyramidal layer: which contains large pyramidal neurons and is the principal source of subcortical efferents.

Multiform cell layer: which contains few large pyramidal neurons and a mixture of small pyramidal and stellate neurons. Layer VI sends efferent fibers to the thalamus, establishing a very precise reciprocal interconnection between the cortex and the thalamus [15].

Pyramidal cell axons in layers III and V contribute to efferent projections that extend to other regions of the CNS. Pyramidal neurons in layer V of the motor cortices send projections all the way down to motor neurons in the spinal cord. Layers I through III are the main target of interhemispheric corticocortical afferents, and layer III is the principal source of corticocortical efferents.

Neuron membranes exhibit a resting potential of approximately -70 millivolts (mV) due to the unequal distribution of sodium ions and potassium ions on the two sides of the nerve cell membrane. The inside of the membrane is negative with respect to the outside [16]. A sodium-potassium pump actively transports three sodium ions out for every two potassium ions transported in, thus establishing the -70 mV resting membrane potential [17].

In addition to the sodium-potassium pump, the nerve cell membrane also contains channels specific for either sodium or potassium ions that allow the respective ions to diffuse through the cell membrane. When the membrane is at rest, sodium channels are closed while some potassium channels are open. Overall there are relatively large amounts of positively charged potassium ions just inside the membrane. On the outside, there are many positively charged sodium ions plus a few potassium ions. When the membrane is stimulated sodium channels are opened causing sodium to diffuse rapidly into the cell along its concentration gradient. This in turn causes the membrane potential to change from -70 mV to +30 mV. This process is known as an action potential. The sodium channels open only briefly after which they close. Afterwards, potassium channels open allowing potassium ions to diffuse outside along a concentration gradient, re-establishing the resting membrane potential [18].

Action potentials only occur when the membrane is depolarized enough so that sodium channels open up completely. A stimulus causes a few sodium channels to open and allows some positively-charged sodium ions to diffuse in. If the membrane potential reaches the threshold potential, voltage-regulated sodium channels all open. Sodium ions rapidly diffuse inward and depolarization occurs. An action potential occurs in an all-or-none fashion and affects only a small area of the nerve cell membrane. The action potential is propagated along the cell membrane through a process known as impulse conduction. For a split second, areas of membrane adjacent to each other have opposite charges causing an electrical circuit to develop between oppositely charged areas. This electrical circuit stimulates the adjacent area causing another action potential. This process repeats itself down the axon nerve cell membrane. This movement of action potentials along a nerve cell is known as an impulse [18].

Impulses travel along a neuron at a velocity from 1 to 120 meters per second. Variation in velocity is determined by fiber diameter and whether or not myelin is present. Neurons with myelin conduct impulses much faster than neurons without myelin. Within the CNS, the myelin sheath is produced by oligodendrocytes. These sheetlike membrane extensions form internodes separated from other internodes by a gap known as a node of Ranvier. Due to the high concentration of sodium channels at the node as well as high electrical resistance within the myelin sheath, action potentials jump from node to node enhancing impulse velocity [18].

Pre-synaptic neuron membranes do not directly contact post-synaptic neuron membranes. An impulse is transmitted to another neuron through the release of chemical neurotransmitters packaged within synaptic vesicles at the end of the axonal bulb. When an impulse arrives at the axonal bulb, the membrane becomes more permeable to calcium enabling calcium to diffuse through the membrane. This activates enzymes that cause synaptic vesicles to move toward the synaptic cleft, fuse with the membrane, and then release neurotransmitter. The neurotransmitter molecules diffuse across the synaptic cleft and bind onto postsynaptic receptor sites, causing physiological responses that may be excitatory or inhibitory depending on the neurotransmitter and receptor type. Residual neurotransmitter molecules are then either pumped back into the presynaptic nerve terminal *via* transporters, destroyed by enzymes, or diffuse into the surrounding area [18].

Neurotransmitters are endogenous chemicals which amplify, relay, and modulate signals between a neuron and another cell. They are packaged into synaptic vesicles that cluster deep to the membrane on the presynaptic side of a synapse, from which they are released into the synaptic cleft. From there, neurotransmitters bind to receptors in the membrane on the postsynaptic side of the synapse. Release of neurotransmitters usually is triggered by the arrival of an impulse at the synapse, but may follow graded electrical potentials. Low level release also occurs without electrical stimulation [19].

Neurotransmitters can be divided into the following types: amino acids, peptides, and monoamines. Examples of amino acid neurotransmitters include: glutamate, aspartate, glycine, serine, NMDA (N-methyl-D-aspartate), and GABA (gamma aminobutyric acid). Monoamines include dopamine, norepinephrine, epinephrine, serotonin, melatonin, and histamine. In addition, over 50 other neuroactive peptides have been found. Examples of other types of neurotransmitters include: ACh (acetylcholine), nitric oxide, adenosine, and anandamide. A few gaseous molecules such as NO (nitric oxide) and CO (carbon monoxide) as well as ions, such as synaptically released zinc, are also considered neurotransmitters.

By far the most prevalent neurotransmitter is glutamate, which is used at well over 90% of the synapses in the human brain [21]. The next most prevalent is GABA, which is used at more than 90% of the synapses that don't use glutamate. Note, however, that even though other transmitters are used in far fewer synapses, they may be very important functionally.

Excitatory neurotransmitters make the postsynaptic membrane less negative by binding with receptor sites and triggering sodium channels to open. This allows an inward diffusion of sodium ions. Subsequently, the membrane potential becomes less negative and approaches the threshold potential. If enough neurotransmitter is released, and enough sodium channels are opened, the membrane potential will reach threshold. If so, an action potential occurs and spreads along the membrane of the post-synaptic neuron allowing signal propagation to continue. Glutamate and aspartate are the major excitatory neurotransmitters in the human central nervous system [20].

Inhibitory neurotransmitters make the postsynaptic membrane potential more negative by binding with receptor sites and triggering an increased permeability to potassium. This decreases the probability of transmission of an impulse from one neuron to another. GABA is a main inhibitory neurotransmitter in the human central nervous system [21, 22].

Any discussion of epileptogenesis without mentioning neurotransmitter receptors would be incomplete, as these receptors play a critical role in both seizure induction and treatment. Excitatory neurotransmitters receptor subtypes include postsynaptic kainate, AMPA, N-methyl-D-aspartate (NMDA), and metabotropic receptors. NMDA and kainate receptors are highly enriched in the hippocampus, an area implicated in the generation of several types of seizures [20].

Excitatory neurotransmitter receptors are associated with a cation channel that opens in response to agonist binding. This allows the cell to depolarize. One specific example of this is involves agonist binding to the NMDA receptor. When this occurs, the resulting partial membrane depolarization removes magnesium blockade of the cation channel. The receptor then acts as an ionophore allowing entry of both extracellular calcium and sodium, causing depolarization. When an agonist binds to the glutamate receptor, calcium is liberated from intracellular stores such as the endoplasmic reticulum initiating a metabolic cascade [20].

Calcium communicates between intracellular organelles in a manner analogous to that of hormones sending intercellular messages. The elevated intracellular calcium leads to activation of numerous enzymes. Calcium ions bind to and activate calmodulin which then becomes a messenger and a regulator of calcium dependent enzymes. Calmodulin in turn activates type II calcium/calmodulin-dependent kinase (CaM Kinase II), which modulates neurotransmitter release through vesicle-membrane interaction, synaptic function, neuronal excitability, and cytoskeletal architecture. CaM Kinase II is highly concentrated in the hippocampus, a site implicated in the development of several types of seizures [23].

Other calcium-dependent pathways also exist. Elevated intracellular calcium is associated with increased phospholipase A2 activity. This leads to production of arachidonic acid, which in turn inhibits glial cell uptake of glutamate intensifying the effect of this excitatory amino acid. Astrocytes also exhibit a form of excitability based on changes of intracellular calcium concentration. Elevated levels of calcium in astrocytes caused the cells to release of the excitatory neurotransmitter glutamate which then can modulate synaptic transmission and neuronal excitability with the nervous system [24].

Elevated extracellular calcium can be problematic. In a small case series study, seizures were associated with calcium carbonate overuse in two patients who had no risk factors for the development of epilepsy. Both eventually developed complex partial seizures correlated with hypercalcemia and were found to have mesial temporal sclerosis on MRI [25].

With regards to inhibitory receptors, an important subtype responds to the neurotransmitter GABA. There are two classes: GABA$_A$ and GABA$_B$. GABA$_A$ receptors are ligand-gated ion channels classified as ionotropic receptors [26]. GABA$_B$ are G protein-coupled receptors classified as metabotropic receptors [27]. The binding of a GABA molecule to an extracellular GABA$_A$ receptor induces a conformational change and opening of a chloride ion-selective channel. This subsequently leads to an influx of chloride which hyperpolarizes the membrane. This action inhibits the firing of new action potentials [26]. The GABA$_A$ also contains a variety of distinc sites that recognize substances such as benzodiazepines, barbituarates, neurosteroids, and ethanol. Benzodiazepines increase the frequency of GABA$_A$ receptor opening whereas barbiturates increase the duration of GABA$_A$ receptor opening.

The GABA$_B$ receptor belongs to a family of G-protein coupled receptors. Though they are located on both presynaptic and postsynaptic membranes, many G-proteins are located on the presynaptic axonal membrane; thus, their activation represents a mechanism of presynaptic inhibition [28, 29]. GABA binding to the presynaptic GABA$_B$ receptor leads to a reduction in the duration of the presynaptic action potential which in turn leads to a reduction in neurotransmitter release [30]. There are two subtypes designated as GABA$_{B1}$ GABA$_{B2}$ [31]. They appear to assemble as heterodimers in neuronal membranes. It is speculated that GABA binding to the receptor induces the two subunits to swing shut around the agonist [32]. The mechanism of action is either from an increase in axonal membrane conductance or from a reduction in voltage-gated calcium channel opening. Either of these changes would reduce the amount of calcium entering the presynaptic terminal causing a corresponding reduction in the amount of transmitter release. Selective agonists at the GABA$_B$ receptor include baclofen, gamma-hydroxybutyrate, phenibut, and 2-aminopropylphosphinic acid. Antagonists include saclofen, phaclofen, and phenylethylamine.

TRANSMISSION OF SEIZURE ACTIVITY FROM THE CEREBRAL CORTEX

To understand how seizure activity within the cerebral cortex causes clinically apparent seizures, a fundamental knowledge of the motor pathways that lead to clinically apparent muscle movement is essential. The corticospinal and corticobulbar tracts play a role in the transmission of seizure activity from the cerebral cortex [33]. Stereotactic neurosurgery cases confirm that in at least some cases abnormal anatomical tissue in the cerebral cortex correlates well with the site of seizure abnormality. Removing the respective portion of the cerebral cortex where the seizures originate can often result in either elimination of seizures or a significant reduction in seizure frequency [34].

Several techniques can be utilized to correlate clinically apparent seizure activity with what is actually happening in the brain. EEG (electroencephalogram) electrodes placed directly on the brain surface of seizure patients can show abnormal neuron cell firing. Two useful imaging techniques include MRI (magnetic resonance imaging) and PET (positron emission tomography). MRI reveals details about brain structure, while PET reveals metabolic activity within the brain. A PET image can show over-activity in the affected part of the brain when taken during seizure activity. Superimposing and combining detailed three-dimensional MRI imaging with PET scan brain activity data gives a representation and correlation of the anatomy and activity within the seizure patient's brain [35].

The corticospinal tract is the main tract for voluntary muscle activity in the body. Although originally thought to only arise exclusively from the precentral gyrus of the frontal lobe, recent studies have shown that it can arise from the postcentral gyrus as well [36]. Large pyramid-shaped neuron cell bodies are located within the precentral gyrus. Axons leave the cortex and pass down through the internal capsule. The axon fibers then proceed into the basis pedunculi of the midbrain and continue down the brainstem into the medulla oblongata. Here 80-90 percent of the axons decussate to the opposite side of the medulla and then descend down the spinal cord. These fibers are situated in the lateral white columns of the cord and are thus called the lateral corticospinal tract. The few axons that do not cross over in the medulla continue down on the ipsilateral side to enter the ventral white columns of the spinal cord. They therefore are known as the ventral corticospinal tract [37].

At each corresponding level of the spinal cord, axons from the lateral corticospinal tract redirect and enter the gray matter of the ventral horn where they synapse with second-order neurons also known as lower motor neurons. At each corresponding level of the spinal cord axons of the ventral corticospinal tract redirect and cross over to the contralateral side of the ventral horn where they also terminate with lower motor neurons [37].

The corticobulbar tract is the main tract for voluntary muscle activity in the head. As with the corticospinal tract, the corticobulbar tract is a two-neuron pathway consisting of an upper motor neuron originating in the cerebral cortex. The upper motor neuron axon synapses with a lower motor neuron. The cell bodies of lower motor neurons of the corticobulbar tract are located within specific areas of the brainstem called nuclei. The axons of these lower motor neurons form many of the cranial nerves [37].

GENERAL PRINCIPLES OF NEUROTOXICOLOGY

Before a toxic agent can reach the CNS and initiate a chain of events that eventually manifest as clinical seizures, it must first enter the body and then bypass the various defense or chemical clearance mechanisms of the body. The effects of a toxic agent can be immediate or delayed. Whether or not the effect of such an agent is reversible depends on whether the agent causes transient changes, permanent changes such as cell death, and on the ability of the damaged cells to recover or regenerate. Cells of the nervous system have limited capacity to regenerate and are less likely to recover after injury relative to other cell types in the body.

The probability that a chemical will enter the body usually depends on the duration, intensity and frequency of chemical exposure and the ability of the chemical to be absorbed by the given route(s) of exposure. Once a toxic substance is absorbed, it will go through some or all of the following processes: distribution, metabolism, and excretion [38]. The severity of cell injury is usually related to the concentration of the toxic substances at its site of action, which in turn is determined by the bioavailability or the extent to which the substance reaches its site of action. The route that a toxic substance enters the body can determine the relative bioavailability of that substance at its site of action, such as the brain. For example, when cyanide is ingested orally, it is absorbed and undergoes hepatic metabolism. However, if the cyanide gas is absorbed through the pulmonary circulation, it travels directly to the brain.

Absorption, distribution, metabolism, and excretion involve passage of toxic substances through cell membranes. Such membrane permeability is dependent upon a toxic substance's molecular size and shape, degree of ionization, and lipid solubility. The rate of absorption is dependent upon the solubility and concentration of the toxic substance. Agents in aqueous solution are more rapidly absorbed than those in oily suspension. Absorption is increased at sites that have relatively more blood flow or large absorptive surface areas such as the lung or gastrointestinal tract. Ingested toxic substances are often absorbed in the small intestine. Inhaled gaseous and toxic substances may be absorbed through the pulmonary epithelium in the respiratory tract. Because the surface area of the lung is so large and blood flow is great, access to circulation is rapid. Absorption of gases is dependent upon their solubility. Highly water-soluble gases are absorbed in the upper airways causing marked irritation and therefore an early warning sign. Toxic gases of low water solubility have few early warning signs and thus reach the lungs. Certain toxic substances can pass through skin as well. The amount of absorption is proportionate to the surface area of contact and to the agent's lipid solubility. Chemicals can also enter the body through ocular absorption by traversing the conjunctiva [38].

Once absorbed toxic substances are transported *via* the blood stream to various areas of the body after which they are distributed into interstitial and cellular fluids. Cardiac output and regional blood flow usually determines the initial phase of distribution. Distribution may be limited by binding of toxic substances to plasma proteins. Toxic agents can accumulate to higher concentrations in tissue as a result of pH gradients, partitioning into lipids, or binding to special cellular proteins. Some agents accumulate in tissue reservoirs and may have prolonged effects.

Lipid soluble toxic substances may be biotransformed into more polar products to enhance removal by urinary excretion. The most common site for biotransformation is the liver. It can also occur in the lungs, in plasma, and other tissues. In some cases biotransformation may result in detoxification, while in other cases it may result in activating or enhancing the toxicity of a compound. Hepatic biotransformation occurs by hydrolysis, oxidation, reduction, and conjugation [38]. Microsomal enzymes are critical in the process. The activity of microsomal enzymes may be induced by environmental or pharmacologic agents. Individual variability in microsomal enzyme activity is genetically determined and accounts for the marked variability in bioavailability of toxic substances. Since many hepatic metabolic systems are not fully developed in neonates, they may be much more susceptible to toxic substances. Individuals with hepatic failure may also be more susceptible due to compromised hepatic metabolic ability.

After a toxic substance has been biotransformed into a polar product it is removed through urinary excretion by the kidney. Renal excretion involves glomerular filtration, secretion, and passive tubular reabsorption [38]. Toxic substances can also be excreted in the bile, sweat, saliva, breast milk, and through the lungs.

Toxic substances or metabolites that bypass excretion, first traverse a unique semi-permeable membrane known as the blood-brain barrier (BBB) prior to entry into the CNS. The BBB is a separation between circulating blood and CSF (cerebrospinal fluid). It is composed of tightly packed endothelial cells that restrict the diffusion of microscopic particles, hydrophilic molecules, and large molecules into the CSF, while allowing the diffusion of small hydrophobic molecules [39]. Thus the BBB is often the rate-limiting factor in determining permeation of substances into the brain. Specific proteins within the BBB actively transport molecules such as glucose from the bloodstream into the CNS. Astrocytes form a layer around brain blood vessels providing biochemical support and may be responsible for transporting ions from the brain to the blood.

The fetal and neonatal BBB is not very mature or effective, and thus are more prone to allowing toxic substances to enter the CNS. The BBB can also be compromised under medical conditions such as hypertension, trauma, ischemia, and inflammation, and hyperosmolality, which can open up the BBB. Both ionizing radiation and non-ionizing radiation can also open the BBB [39].

The BBB can be bypassed at natural gate points known as circumventricular organs (CVOs) where relatively large molecular weight and polar substances can pass back and forth from blood to the perivascular space. CVOs are structures that border ventricular spaces in the midline of the brain. Unlike other areas in the brain, glial cells within

CVOs are loosely apposed creating relatively large perivascular spaces. Additionally, the tight junctions between endothelial cells lining these vessels are nonexistent. Therefore CVOs are in cellular contact with both blood and CSF and have been termed "windows of the brain". Hypothetically, CVOs serve to relay information among neural cells, CSF, and blood. Special ependymal cells within CVOs called tanycytes communicate throughout the neuroaxis through neural connections with strategic nuclei [40, 41].

Within the ventricles, modified ependymal cells and capillaries form the choroid plexus which produces the CSF [42]. The CSF essentially has open communication with the extracellular fluid (ECF) surrounding the neurons and support cells of the CNS. CSF has been described as a reservoir of cerebral ECF, and is housed by the ventricles in the brain and the central canal of the spinal cord [41]. The concentrations of substances within the CSF inside the ventricular system can vary by a factor of 10 in different regions of the brain [43].

CSF is held within the brain ventricles which are lined by specialized simple cuboidal epithelial cells known as ependymal cells. These cells are layered with cilia on their apical surface which serve to circulate CSF around the CNS. Their apical surfaces also have microvilli that absorb CSF. Between ependymal cells, tight junctions known as zonae occludentes, control CSF release across the epithelium resulting in exchange between CSF and nervous tissue of brain. Neuroactive substances within the CSF flow toward the ECF compartment. The amount of substance that reaches the ECF is variable with concentrations varying over time. Large regional concentration differences have been observed for such substances [44- 45].

Exchange of fluid contents between the nervous tissue ECF and ventricular CSF is known to occur *via* three different mechanisms: diffusion, perivascular pump mechanisms, and internalization by tanycytes and neurons in direct contact with CSF [43]. Due to the lack of tight junctions between ependymal cells, diffusion and exchange between CSF and ECF compartments may occur in both directions through the uninterrupted single-layered lining of the ventricular system.

Perivascular pumps distribute CSF contents into deeper tissues of the brain. Such pumps are created by penetration of the outer brain surface by the perivascular space around vessels. Arterial pulsations of the cerebral vessels drive the pump [46, 47]. Perivascular pumps play an important role in distributing substances within the brain.

Special ependymal cells (tanycytes) and neurons in direct contact with CSF internalize specific constituents and release them at specific targeted sites within the brain [48]. Certain neurons have also been observed to exhibit selective receptor-mediated uptake of substances from the CSF.

CSF departs the CNS through three main routes. Approximately one third of the CSF leaves *via* the spinal vessels, one third *via* the nasal lymphatics, and about one third is absorbed through arachnoid granulations into the superior sagittal sinus [43, 49-50].

MECHANISMS OF CHEMICALLY INDUCED SEIZURES AND EPILEPTOGENESIS

Once past the BBB, the substance must diffuse through the CSF flowing through the neuroaxis *via* the ventricular system. From there it is essentially in contact with the ECF around the neural tissue. Ependymal cells and neurons adjacent to the CSF transport the substance to specific sites within the brain. The substance can then exert local effects on the brain tissue it is in direct contact with, which can lead to aberrant electrical activity. If substance exposure repeatedly continues to elicit seizures, eventually the seizures occur spontaneously in a process known as kindling. When such a condition occurs, this is known as epilepsy.

Repeated paroxysmal electrical discharges can cause distant CNS lesions in areas not directly exposed to a seizure-inducing substance. In rat models in which seizures were induced by injection of kainate (KA) into the amygdala, direct toxic damage to the hippocampus was observed as a consequence of KA diffusion from the amygdala to the hippocampus. In the same study diazepam was administered to limit electrical discharges. This blocked distant damage to the hippocampus even in the presence of direct damage to the amygdala by KA. Collectively these findings show indirectly that distant damage to the hippocampus is also mediated by aberrant electrical discharges and not merely by direct toxic effects occurring after KA had time to diffuse to the hippocampus [51].

In recurrent epileptic seizures, aberrant sprouting and synaptic reorganization of mossy fiber (MF) axons are often found in the hippocampus of temporal lobe epilepsy patients. Studies on *ex vivo* hippocampus cultures show that prolonged hyperactivity induces MF sprouting as well as neural network reorganization. Brain-derived neurotrophic factor (BDNF) has been implicated as the causal agent of MF sprouting. Hyperexcitation induces upregulation of BDNF expression, which in turn induces MF axonal branching. The newly sprouted branches are then ectopically guided into the deeper molecular layer where they synapse with dendrites of granule cells. Such abnormal recurrent circuits cause hyperexcitation of the dentate gyrus [4- 6].

Epileptogenesis, or the occurrence of spontaneous seizures, hypothetically occurs when a seizure-inducing substance triggers a range of molecular, structural, and functional changes. Large scale genomic studies have shown changes in hundreds of genes shortly after status epilepticus. Many of these genes are associated with gliosis, neuronal death, neurogenesis, neuronal plasticity, and structural reorganization [4-6, 52]. Therefore, many genes likely contribute to seizure induction and the loss of synaptic plasticity observed in epilepsy.

Waves of gene induction have been observed. Genes belonging to specific processes are often induced or repressed at certain points in time during epileptogenesis. Rat models show that in early acute stages, biological processes appear to be related to transcriptional and translational processes involved in short-term stress response to seizure activity. Such changes were associated with cell death and local tissue inflammatory reaction. Genes related to the immune response and apoptosis were also enhanced [52- 53]. At the same time, genes related to processes associated with synaptic transmission, synaptic plasticity, calcium homeostasis, and cell adhesions were repressed. In the latent phase, genes expression related to the immune and inflammatory response, antigen processing, response to injury, and lysosome production became prominent. In the chronic phase, important gene expression processes include acute phase response and intracellular protein transport [52]. CaMK-associated genes were downregulated. Downregulation of CaMKIIalpha has been correlated to neuronal cell death, hyperexcitability, and epilepsy [54-56]. Calcium- and calmodulin- dependent protein kinase activity were downregulated as well. GABA receptor subunits were downregulated significantly both acutely and chronically, while glutamate signaling-related genes were downregulated acutely but had recovered after the latent period [52].

In the same rat model, the immune response was the most prominent process changed during the phases leading up to epileptogenesis. Prostaglandin synthesis was activated, which in turn increases intracellular calcium and subsequent glutamate release. This in turn would increases excitability in surrounding neural networks. Complement activation also occurs. Intrusion of brain tissue by immune system components such as monocytes and neutrophils might also play a role in destabilizing surrounding networks [52].

Neurons are not the only cell types involved in seizure induction. Glial cells also likely contribute to epileptogenesis. In animal models, a large number of glial genes are maximally expressed 1 week after seizure induction. Such genes are linked to the immune and inflammatory response as well as genes related to ion homeostasis. Repression of ion transport *via* down regulation of potassium, sodium and calcium channels, and glial redistribution of water channels involved in water homeostasis could lead to increased excitability. This data correlates to several studies in which glutamate released from glial cells activates NMDA receptors causing a slow inward current in nearby neurons, which could possibly caused synchronized neural activity. Experimental models of focal cortical epilepsy have shown that glial pathology is a universal feature of focal epilepsy. Hypertrophied astrocytes have been observed before seizure development. One study concluded that astrocytes can generate paroxysmal depolarization shifts in neurons through release of glutamate, even in the absence of synaptic interactions among neurons [52].

Genetic studies have yielded additional information as well. In *Drosophila melanogaster* genetic studies, mutant species more prone to seizures were determined to possess a mutant seizure locus that structurally altered voltage-sensitive sodium channels [57].

A critical gene change observed after seizure activity is the consistent down regulation of genes encoding for subunits of extrasynaptic receptors that control tonic inhibition. Such impaired tonic inhibition can lead to dynamic disturbance of neuronal networks and subsequent epileptiform oscillations [52].

Other changes observed in animal model cells exposed to stress or seizure damage are an immediate increased expression of early response genes (ERGs) that code for transcription factors, receptors, kinases and cytokines resulting in alteration of cellular physiology [53].

In other studies, hexahydro-1,3,5-trinitro-1,3,5-triazine (RDX) induced seizures in certain bird species. Comparative toxicology shows a similarity between RDX-induced seizures in birds and organochlorine insecticide dichlorodiphenyltrichloroethane (DDT)-induced seizures in mammals in regards to molecular mechanisms. DDT neurotoxicity in mammals causes a delayed repolarization of neuron postaction potential leading to hyperexcitability. In the DDT seizure response, several underlying mechanisms were observed: 1) Reduced potassium transport across the neuronal membrane 2) slowed closing of sodium channels postaction potential 3) inhibition of calmodulin control of calcium at axonal nodes triggering neurotransmitter release and 4) inhibition of neuronal sodium, potassium, and calcium ATPases. Sodium and potassium ATPases are necessary to drive active transport of sodium and potassium against concentration gradients to reestablish repolarization of neuron membranes [58].

RDX possibly elicits seizures through inhibition of the neuronal cell repolarization postaction potential leading to heightened neuronal excitability and seizures. RDX-induced seizures occurred in a dose-dependent manner. Birds exposed to RDX that had seizures accumulated over 20 times more RDX in their brain tissue than RDX exposed birds that did not have seizures despite a common dose exposure level. Since the BBB does not effectively exclude RDX from brain tissue, RDX-non-seizing birds must have metabolized RDX extensively as indicated by the lower levels of RDX in liver tissue reflecting the critical importance of detoxification and excretion to prevent accumulation of RDX in CNS tissue [58].

Tissue RDX-levels were correlated directly with impacts on gene expression and seizures. Within the RDX-seizing birds, differentially expressed genes have gene ontology functions associated with cell signaling and electrophysiology within the CNS. The differentially expressed genes are involved in functions such as calcium signaling, cell communication, ion transport, and metal ion biding. Conversely, RDX-non-seizing birds and controls (unexposed to RDX) displayed little difference in overall transcript expression relative to transcript targets identified to be significantly affected by RDX exposure in RDX-seizing birds [58].

Seizure disorders are genetically complex. As shown in the RDX bird experiment, the ability to detoxify and excrete a chemical before it can reach the BBB and elicit a seizure is genetically determined. In mice experiments involving the seizure-inducing chemical pentylenetetrazol (PTZ), a certain genotype was found to be more susceptible to PTZ-induced-seizures relative to another. The location of genes responsible for such differential sensitivity was mapped to particular loci. PTZ blocks GABA receptors in the brain. Interestingly, KA-induced-seizures are caused by activation of glutamate receptors. Genes responsible for susceptibility to KA have also been mapped to particular loci. Possibly, a genetic locus that affects the function of the two main neurotransmitter systems in the CNS may play a critical role in the final common pathway for regulating neuronal excitability.

Substances can exert direct physical effect or damage locally on neurons through various mechanisms which include: 1) ion channels disruption 2) enhancement of synaptic transmission of excitatory neurotransmitters 3) increase in intracellular calcium 4) interference with neurotransmitter receptors through inhibition of GABA receptor function or enhancement of excitatory neurotransmitter receptor function such as at NMDA receptors or 5) paroxysmal discharge. As more seizure activity occurs, damage can also occur distally along the circuit pathway even in areas not directly exposed to a toxic substance..

In the case of temporal lobe epilepsy, anatomic and cellular alterations occur in the dentate gyrus of the hippocampus. In most cases, the granule cell layer is preserved, but is dispersed with ectopic granule neurons observed in the hilus and inner molecular layer. The dentate granular cells also give rise to abnormal axonal projections to the supragranular inner molecular layer in a process known as mossy fiber "sprouting". These aberrant connections formed by newly born dentate granule cells may lead to hippocampal network plasticity associated with epileptogenesis.

MODELS AND EXAMPLES OF SEIZURES CAUSED BY SPECIFIC CHEMICALS

Numerous chemicals are known to induce seizure activity. A few select examples will be discussed, the first of which are the organophosphorus (OP) nerve agents designed for warfare. Examples include sarin, soman, and *O-*

Ethyl *S*-(2-diisopropylaminoethyl) methylphosphonothioate (VX). If unchecked these nerve agents irreversibly inhibit acetylcholinesterase (AchE) in both the CNS and PNS, resulting in excess acetylcholine stimulation. Thus, nerve agent exposure is typically treated with an anticholinergic such as atropine and an oxime such as pyridine-2-aldoxime methycloride (2-PAM) to reactive inhibited AchE [59-60]. One study found that central muscarinic cholinergic mechanisms are involved in eliciting early seizures following exposure to soman [61]. Studies in which animals were exposed to soman have shown that seizures typically do not occur unless AchE inhibition reaches at least 65% [62]. Because the initial seizure activity caused by OP nerve agents is cholinergic in nature, anticholinergics readily terminate seizures and prevent neuropathology at this early stage of exposure. However, if not given soon enough a transition phase occurs during which the neuronal seizure activity perturbs other neurotransmitter systems. Excitatory amino acid levels increase and contribute to seizure activity. One such amino acid is glutamate which plays a prominent role in the maintenance of OP-induced seizures through over-activation of NMDA receptors [63]. Changes in inhibitory GABA activity in brain regions enriched with cholinergic inputs such as the hippocampus, also contribute to the maintenance of OP-induced seizures [64]. At this intermediate stage, anticholinergics become less effective. Eventually seizure activity enters a phase in which anticholinergics are no longer effective. In this latter phase, NMDA antagonists remain effective as anticonvulsants when co-administered with anticholinergics [65]. When seizure activity in sarin exposed rats was limited by treatment with midazolam 5 minutes after exposure, no prolonged seizure activity or release of inflammatory markers was observed. When midazolam treatment was withheld until 30 minutes after exposure, prolonged seizures occurred and inflammatory markers were increased even 30 days following sarin exposure [66].

Recently galantamine has received much attention as a potential antidote to prevent OP-induced seizures. Galantamine is a reversible competitive AchE inhibitor and an allosteric modulator of nicotinic AchRs [67, 68]. Soman exposure reduces inhibitory postsynaptic current (IPSC) frequency in pyramidal neurons of guinea pigs, contributing to excess neuronal discharge. Pretreatment of guinea pigs with galantamine prevents the effect of soman on IPSCs within the hippocampus. Gacyclidine (GK-11), a non-competitive NMDA antagonist, has also been shown to be effective in preventing OP-induced seizures when it is given prior to OP exposure or immediately after exposure [69]. In summary, various antidotes to prevent or minimize OP induced seizures and permanent neuropathology work at different stages due to various mechanisms of seizure induction. Treatment must be initiated immediately to prevent a cascade of events that will lead to irreversible neurological damage and prolonged clinical seizure.

Chemicals that induce cerebral hypoxia can also elicit seizure activity. Such chemicals include carbon monoxide (CO) and cyanide, although the two cause hypoxia *via* different mechanisms. CO reversibly binds to hemoglobin 230-270 times stronger than to oxygen. Thus even at small concentrations it can displace relatively large amounts of oxygen and cause a functional anemia. Additionally, binding of CO to hemoglobin causes an increased binding of oxygen at the remaining oxygen-binding sites, further decreasing oxygen delivery to already compromised hypoxic tissues. CO also binds to cytochrome c oxydase resulting in interference with aerobic metabolism and ATP synthesis. Cells switch to anaerobic metabolism which leads to anoxia, lactic acidosis, and cell death [69, 70].

Cyanide in salt or solid form can be absorbed from the gastrointestinal tract if orally ingested. The cyanide salt combines with stomach acid to release gas. Although cyanide can be absorbed through intact skin, this route of entry typically is not of clinical significance. The most important route of entry under battlefield conditions would be through inhalation. Following absorption, cyanide is rapidly distributed all organs and tissues of the body. Both ingestion and inhalation lead to high concentrations in the brain. The cyanide ion rapidly combines with iron in cytochrome a_3 to inhibit this enzyme. This in turn leads to a chain of events that prevent intracellular oxygen utilization. Within 30 seconds of inhalation, clinically apparent seizures begin [71].

Regardless of the specific etiological mechanism, cerebral hypoxia causes astrocyte proliferation. These astrocytes do not function normally and result in reversal of glutamate uptake [72]. Presynaptic membrane ion pumps and calcium-mediated exocytosis is thought to contribute to release of glutamate from neurons [73-75]. Additionally, hypoxia causes changes in both AMPA and NMDA glutamate receptors. This leads to increased free intracellular calcium and neuronal hyperexcitability [72].

There are many more examples of chemicals that elicit seizure activity; however, their discussion is beyond the scope of this chapter. Suffice to say that due to the myriad of mechanisms through which substances can cause seizures and in some cases epilepsy, it follows that there are potentially numerous ways to not only suppress seizures, but to prevent seizures and progression to epilepsy. Further research and understanding of seizure mechanisms will likely lead to discovery of methods by which to treat and ultimately prevent seizure or epilepsy development. The interaction of multiple genes products likely leads to epilepsy. Knowledge of predisposing genes will help in the development of therapeutics.

REFERENCES

[1]   University of Maryland Medical Center. Epilepsy – causes. http://www.umm.edu/patiented/articles/what_causes_of_epilepsy_000044_2.htm. (accessed Dec 2, 2009).

[2]   Fisher RS, Boas WV, Blume W. Epileptic Seizures and Epilepsy: Definitions Proposed by the International League Against Epilepsy (ILAE) and the International Bureau for Epilepsy (IBE). Epilepsia 2005; 46: 470-2.

[3]   Bertrum E. The relevance of kindling for human epilepsy. Epilepsia 2007; S2: 65-74.

[4]   Koyama R, Yamada MK, Fijisawa S, *et al.* Brain-derived neurotrophic factor induces hyperexcitable reentrant circuits in the dentate gyrus. J Neurosci 2004; 24: 7215-24.

[5]   Parent JM, Yu TW, Leibowitz RT, *et al.* Dentate granule cell neurogenesis is increased by seizures and contributes to aberrant network reorganization in the adult rate hippocampus. J Neurosci 1997; 17(10): 3727-38.

[6]   Sutula T, Koch J, Golarai G, *et al.* NMDA receptor dependence of kindling and mossy fiber sprouting: evidence that the NMDA receptor regulates patterning of hippocampal circuits in the adult brain. Journal Neurosci 1996; 16: 7398-406.

[7]   Julien JP. Neurofilament functions in health and disease. Curr Opin Neurobiol 1999; 9(5): 554-60.

[8]   He Z, Koprivica V. The Nogo signaling pathway for regeneration block. Annu Rev Neurosci, 2004; 2: 341-68.

[9]   Elson GN. Cortex, cognition and the cell: new insights into the pyramidal neuron and prefrontal function. Cereb Cortex 2003; 13: 1124-38.

[10]   Magee J, Hoffman D, Colbert C, *et al.* Electrical and calcium signaling in dendrites of hippocampal pyramidal neurons. Annu Rev Physiol 1998; 60: 327-46.

[11]   Megías M, Emri Z, Freund TF, *et al.* Total number and distribution of inhibitory and excitatory synapses on hippocampal CA1 pyramidal cells. Neurosci 2001; 102: 527–40.

[12]   Azevedo VA, Carvalho LR, Grinberg LT, *et al.* Equal numbers of neuronal and nonneuronal cells make the human brain an isometrically scaled-up primate brain. J Comp Neurol 2009; 513: 532-41.

[13]   Herrup C, Yang Y. Cell cycle regulation in the postmitotic neuron: oxymoron or new biology?. Nature Rev Neurosci, 2007; 8: 368-78.

[14]   Rogawski MA. Astrocytes get in the act in epilepsy. Nat Med 2005; 11: 919-20.

[15]   Shipp S. Structure and function of the cerebral cortex. Curr Biol 2007; 17: R443-9.

[16]   Chudler EH. Lights, camera, action potential: Neuroscience for Kids. http:faculty.Washington.edu/chudler/ap/html (accessed Dec 11, 2009).

[17]   Gregory MJ. The Biology Web: The nervous system: neurons. faculty.clintoncc.suny.edu/faculty/michael.../neurons.htm (accessed Apr 21, 2010).

[18]   Ritchison G. Bio 101 Human Physiology: Neurons & the nervous system.people.eku.edu/ritchisong/301notes2.htm (accessed Dec 11, 2009).

[19]   King MW. The Medical Biochemistry Page: Biochemistry of neurotransmitters. themedicalbiochemistrypage.org/nerves.html (accessed Aug 4, 2010).

[20]   Clark S, Stasheff S, Lewis DV, *et al.* In: JC Watskins, Ed. The NMDA receptor. New York, Oxford University Press 1994; pp. 396-414.

[21]   Meldrum BS. Glutamate as a Neurotransmitter in the Brain: Review of Physiology and Pathology. J Nutr 2000; 130: 1007S-15S.

[22]   Chang Y, Wang R, Barot S, *et al.* Stoichiometry of a recombinant GABAA receptor. J Neurosci 1996; 16: 5415-24.

[23]   Yasui M, Storng MJ, Ota K, *et al.* Mineral and metal neurotoxicology. New York: CRC Press 1997.

[24]   Parpura V, Haydon PG. Physiological astrocyte calcium levels stimulate glutamate release to modulate adjacent neurons. Proc Natl Acad Sci 2000; 97: 8629-34.

[25]   Dinnerstein E, McDonald BC, Cleavinger HB, *et al.* Mesial temporal sclerosis after status epilepticus due to milk alkali syndrome. Seizure 2008; 17: 292-5.

[26]   Hevers W, Luddens H. The diversity of GABAA receptors. Pharmacological and electrophysiological properties of GABAA channel subtypes. Mol Neurobiol 1998; 18: 35-86.

[27]   Chen K, Li H, Ye N, *et al.* Role of GABAB receptors in GABA and baclofen-induced inhibition of adult rat cerebellar interpositus nucleus neurons *in vitro*. Brain Res Bull 2005; 67: 310-8.

[28]   Curtis DR, Hosli L, Johnston GAR, *et al.* The hyperpolarization of spinal motor neurons by glycine and related amino-acids. Exp Brain Res 1968; 5: 235-58.

[29]   Curtis DR, Lodge D, Brand SJ. GABA and spinal afferent terminal excitability in the cat. Brain Res 1977; 130: 360-63.

[30]   Kaupmann K, Hugle K, Heid J, *et al.* Expression cloning of GABAB receptors uncovers similarity to metabotropic glutamate receptors. Nature 1997; 386(6622): 239-46.

[31]   Purves D, Augustine GJ, Fitzpatrick D, *et al.* Neuroscience. 2nd ed. Sunderland: Sinauer Associates, Inc 2001.

[32]   Martin IL, Dunn SMJ. GABA receptors. Bristol: Tocris Cookson Ltd. 2002.

[33]   Sarnat HB. Functions of the corticospinal and corticobulbar tracts in the human newborn. J Ped Neurol 2003; 1: 3-8.

[34]   Mayo Clinic. Epilepsy surgery: Why it's done. http://www.mayoclinic.com/health/epilepsy (accessed Dec 13, 2009).

[35]   MGH News. Surgery for Epilepsy. http://neurosurgery.mgh.harvard.edu/functional/ep-mrcl.htm. (accessed Dec 13, 2009).

[36]   Kumar A, 1-8.Johasz C, Asano E, *et al.* Diffusion tensor imaging study of the cortical origin and course of the corticospinal tract in healthy children. Am J Neuroradiol 2009; 10.3174/ajnr.A1742:

[37]   Liebman M. Neuroanatomy made easy and understandable. 4th ed. Gaithersburg: Aspen Publishers, Inc. 1991.

[38]   Becker CE, Rosenberg J. In: LaDou J, Ed. Occupational medicine. Norwalk, Appleton & Lange 1990; pp. 131-139.

[39]   Scott RM. Chemical hazards in the workplace. Chelsea, Lewis Publishers, Inc. 1989.

[40]   Johnson AK, Gross PM. Sensory circumventricular organs and brain homeostatic pathways. FASEB J 1993; 7: 678-86.

[41]   Borson HL, Borison R, McCarthy LE. Brain stem penetration by horseradish peroxidase from the cerebrospinal fluid spaces in the cat. Exp Neurol 1980; 69: 271-89.

[42]   Edsbagge M, Tisell M, Jacobson L, *et al.* Spinal CSF absorption in healthy individuals. Am J Physiol Regul Integr Comp Physiol 2004; 287: R1450-55.

[43]   Veening JG, Berendregt HP. The regulation of brain states by neuroactive substances distributed *via* the cerebrospinal fluid; a review. Cerebrospinal Fluid Res 2010; 7: 1-18.

[44]   Reiber H. Proteins in cerebrospinal fluid and blood: barriers, CSF flow rate and source-related dynamics. Restor Neurol Neurosci 2003; 21: 79-96.

[45]   Tricoire H, Moller M, Chemineau P, *et al.* Origin of cerebrospinal fluid melatonin and possible function in the integration of photoperiod. Reprod Suppl 2003; 61: 311-21.

[46]   Renneis ML, Gregory TF, Blaumanis OR, *et al.* Evidence for a 'paravascular' fluid circulation in the mammalian central nervous system, provided by the rapid distribution of tracer protein throughout the brain from the subarachnoid space. Brain Res 1985; 326: 47-63.

[47]   Hadaczek P, Yamashita Y, Mirek H, *et al.* The "perivascular pump" driven by arterial pulsation is a powerful mechanism for the distribution of therapeutic molecules within the brain. Mol Ther 2006; 14: 69-78.

[48]   Rodriguez EM, Blazquez JL, Pastor FE, *et al.* Hypothalamic tanycytes: a key component of brain-endocrine interaction. Int Rev Cytol 2005; 247: 89-164.

[49]   Maillot C: The perispinal spaces. Constitution, organization, and relations with the cerebrospinal fluid (CSF). J Neuroradiol 1991; 18: 18-31.

[50]   Johnston M, Armstron D, Koh L. Possible role of cavernous sinus veins in cerebrospinal fluid absorption. Cerebrospinal Fluid Res 2007; 4: 3.

[51]   Lee MC, Ban SS, Woo YJ, *et al.* Calcium/calmodulin kinase II activity of hippocampus in kainite-induced epilepsy. J Korean Med Sci 2001; 16: 643-8.

[52]   Gorter JA, van Vliet EA, Aronica E, *et al.* Potential new antiepileptic targets indicated by microarray analysis in a rat model for temporal lobe epilepsy. J Neurosci 2006; 26: 11083-110.

[53]   Westmark CJ, Gourronc FA, Bartleson VB, *et al.* HuR mRNA ligands expressed after seizure. J Neuropathol Exp Neurol 2005; 64: 1037-45.

[54]   Butler LS, Silva AJ, Abeliovich A, *et al.* Limbic epilepsy in transgenic mice carrying a Ca2+/calmodulin kinase II alpha-subunit mutation. Proce Natl Acad Sci 1995; 92: 6852-55.

[55]   Churn SB, Kochan LD, DeLorenzo RJ. Chronic inhibition of Ca2+/calmodulin kinase II activity in the pilocarpine model of epilepsy. Brain Res 2000; 875: 66-77.

[56]   Simonato M, Bregola G, Armellin M, *et al.* Dendritic targeting of mRNAs for plasticity genes in experimental models of temporal lob epilepsy. Epilepsia 2002; 43: 153-8.

[57]   Jackson RB, Gitchier J, Strichartz GR, *et al.* Genetic modifications of voltage-sensitive sodium channels in Drosophila: gene dosage studies of the seizure locus. J Neurosci 1985; 5: 1144-51.

[58] Gust KA, Pirooznia M, Quinn MJ, *et al.* Neurotoxicogenomic investigations to assess mechanisms of action of the munitions constituents RDX and 2,6-DNT in northern bobwhite (Colinus virginianus). Oxford J 2009; 110: 168-80.

[59] Moore DH, Clifford, CB, Crawford IT, *et al.* In: Quinn DM, Balaubramanian AS, Doctor BP, *et al.*, Eds. Enzymes of the cholinesterase family. New York, Plenum Press 1995; pp. 297-304.

[60] Tylor P. Anticholinesterase agents. In: Hardman JG, Limbird LE, and Gilman AG, Eds. Goodman and Gilman's the pharmacological basis of therapeutics, 10th ed. New York, McGraw-Hill Companies 2001; pp. 110-29.

[61] Shih TM, Koviak TA, Capcio BR. Anticonvulsants for poisoning by the organophosphorus compound soman: pharmogological mechanisms. Neurosci Biobehav Rev 1991; 15: 349-62.

[62] Tonduli LS, Testylier G, Marino IP, *et al.* Triggering of soman-induced seizures in rats: multiparametric analysis with special correlation between enzymatic, neurochemcial, and electrophysiological data. J Neurosci Res 1999; 58: 464-73.

[63] Lallement G, Baubichon D, Clarencon D, *et al.* Review of the value of gacylidine (GK-11) as adjuvant medication to convention treatments of organophosphate poisoning: primate experiments mimicking various scenarios of military or terrorist attack by soman. Neurotox 1999; 20(4): 675-84.

[64] Shih TM, McDonough JH. Neurochemical mechanisms in soman-induced seizures. J Appl Toxicol 1997; 17: 255-64.

[65] McDonough JH, Shih TM. Neuropharmacological mechanisms of nerve agent-induced seizure and neuropathology. Neurosci BioBehav Rev 1997; 21: 559-79.

[66] Chapman S, Kadar T, Gilat E. Seizure duration following sarin exposure affects neuro-inflammatory markers in the rat brain. Neurotox 2006; 27(2): 277-83.

[67] Maelicke A, Albuquerque EX. Allosteric modulation of nicotinic acetylcholine receptors as a treatment strategy for Alzheimer's disease. Eur J Pharmacol 2000; 393: 165-70.

[68] Pereira ERF, Burt DR, Aracava Y, *et al.* Novel medical countermeasure for organophosphorus intoxication: connection to Alzheimer's disease and dementia. In: Romano JA Jr. Lukey BJ, Salem H, Eds. Chemical warfare agents. Boca Raton, CC Press. 2008: pp. 219-32.

[69] Schochat GN, Lucchesi M. Emergency Medicine: Toxicity, carbon monoxide. http://emedicine.medscape.com/article/819987 (accessed Aug 4, 2010).

[70] Alonso JR, Cardellach F, Lopez S, *et al.* Carbon monoxide specifically inhibits cytochrome c oxidase of human mitochondrial respiratory chain. Pharmacol Toxicol 2003; 93(3):142-46.

[71] United States Army Medical Research Institute of Chemical Defense (USAMRICD). Medical management of chemical casualties handbook, 3rd Ed: Cyanide. www.brooksidepress.org/Products/.../005Cyanide.htm (accessed Aug 28, 2010).

[72] Park EP, Bell JD, Baker AJ. Traumatic brain injury: Can the consequences be stopped? Can Med Assoc J 2008; 178(9): 1163-70.

[73] Taylor CP, Meldrum BS. Na+ channels as targets for neuroprotective drugs. Trends Pharmacol Sci 1995; 16: 309-16.

[74] Dirnagl U, Iadecola C, Moskowitz MA. Pathobiology of ischaemic stroke: an integrated view. Trends Neurosci 1999; 22: 391-7.

[75] Endres M, Dirnagl U. Ischemia and stroke. Adv Exp Med Biol 2002; 513: 455-73.

CHAPTER 2

Seizures Associated with Warfare Nerve Agents: Pathophysiology, Clinical Symptoms and Supportive Interventions

Oleg Dolkart, Ron Ben-Abraham and Avi A Weinbroum[*]

Post Anesthesia Care Unit and Animal Research Laboratory, Tel Aviv Sourasky Medical Center, and the Sackler Faculty of Medicine, Tel Aviv University, Tel Aviv, Israel

Abstract: Until more recently, the effects of exposure to chemical warfare agents were a remote area of clinical practice, which concerned military specialists, microbiologists, and toxicologists. Since the World Trade Center attack in New York City in September 2001, there has been real concern about the possible impact of nerve agents (NA) released by terrorists on civilian population. In the pre- and intra-hospital settings, anesthesiologists have since become more involved in the preparedness of such potential mass casualty events together with administrative officials. The former create protocols to improve casualty rescue, management, and outcome, while the latter building up medical contingents, drilling interventional and logistic protocols and provide early and late medical and psychological life support to the care providers and the population.

Exposure to warfare NA intoxicants can cause brain damage, long-term cognitive and behavioral deficits, and even death. In the acute phase of the intoxication, brain damage is primarily caused by intense seizure activity induced by these agents. Also, hypoxia and asphyxia are associated with seizures; however, these may be pre-terminal conditions.

This review will elaborate in detail pre-hospital and intra-hospital management of NA in terms of seizures. Other aspects of medical and administrative attendance associated with these chaotic situations are reviewed elsewhere and will be refereed accordingly. Pathophysiology and clinical management of current trends of life support will be addressed.

INTRODUCTION

In today's global political climate the use of nerve agents (NA) poses a major threat, both to the soldier or health providers in the frontline as well as to civilian populations. All compounds are relatively simple to produce, transport, and deploy. The most known NA are soman, sarin, cyclosarin, tabun, and VX [1-3]. These organophosphorus compounds are all potent irreversible inhibitors of acetylcholinesterase (AChE) causing massive accumulation of acetylcholine at cholinergic synapses. The result is a cholinergic crisis caused by the overstimulation of muscarinic and nicotinic receptors in the central and peripheral nervous system, including the neuromuscular junction [1-4]. The time-course of NA poisoning is rapid, and death may occur within minutes depending on a number of factors, with the dose and the route of exposure being most important among them [1-3]. Even when death is prevented pharmacologically, or the dose of exposure is sub-lethal, long-lasting neurological and behavioral symptoms may still occur because of damage to the central nervous system [5-11]. However, the characteristic acute neurological deterioration so feared after exposure to NA is primarily due to seizure activity, which can rapidly progress to status epilepticus [11-14]. Convulsions are a major sign of NA poisoning of the CNS [15] and NA-induced seizures rapidly progress to status epilepticus, which leads to profound structural brain damage [16, 17].

Brain seizures after NA exposure are mainly induced by over-stimulation of brain muscarinic receptors [18]. These receptors are widely distributed within the brain, and are located at post-synaptic sites where they mediate excitatory effects of acetylcholine, such as blockade of various potassium conductances [19-22] or activation of calcium-sensitive non-specific cation currents [23]. Also affected are the pre-synaptic terminals that modulate the release of glutamate [24-25] and GABA [26-27]. Consequently, the increased brain levels of glutamate [28-29] and GABA (gamma-amino butyric acid) [30], disrupts the delicate balance in the activity of the two major excitatory and

*Address correspondence to Dr. Avi A. Weinbroum: Post-Anesthesia Care Unit, Tel Aviv Sourasky Medical Center, 6 Weizman St., Tel-Aviv 64239, Israel; Tel: +972-3-6973237; Fax: +972-3-6925749; E-mail: draviw@tasmc.health.gov.il

inhibitory systems in the brain. Thus, cholinergic hyperactivity initiates seizures, which are then perpetuated by the additional triggered glutamatergic hyperactivity. The latter sustains and reinforces brain hyperstimulation and is, eventually, responsible for excitotoxic neuronal damage leading to the long-lasting sequalea after the acute intoxication [18, 28, 31]. Consistent with this view is the clinical observation that central antimuscarinic compounds can reduce or block seizures only when administered within a few minutes after exposure [32- 33].

Several intoxicants can induce seizure activity mainly due to anoxic brain damage as a result of the damage caused to the respiratory system by the intoxication. Such pathological events and their clinical implications are emergency events that are not the purpose of this review.

Recognition of the unique clinical manifestations is the first step in assisting victims of NA occurrence. Careful decontamination and vital supportive care will be the most important steps along with implementing antidotal treatment. This combined antidotal and resuscitation intervention will make the difference in many cases of NA-induced seizures.

NERVE AGENTS

Chemical agents are poisonous vapors, aerosols, gasses, liquids, or solids that have toxic effects on people, animals, or plants. Most of these agents are liquid at room temperature and are disseminated as vapors and aerosols. They may be released as bombs, sprayed from aircraft and boats, or disseminated by other means to intentionally create a hazard to people and the environment. Some of these agents are highly toxic and persistent, features that can render a site uninhabitable and require costly and potentially hazardous decontamination and remediation. Health effects range from irritation and burning of skin and mucous membranes to rapid cardiopulmonary collapse and death.

Decontamination of V agents with hypochlorite can itself produce toxic products and is not recommended. NAs can penetrate clothing, skin, and leather. Rubber and synthetic materials, such as polyethylene and butyl rubber, are more resistant. For further reading regarding secondary intoxication and modes of decontamination see [34- 35].

SEIZURES AND THEIR PATHOPHYSIOLOGY

Seizures are termed generalized or focal OK HERE (partial) depending on their clinical manifestations. The former type of seizure results from the abnormal electrical event that simultaneously involves both cerebral hemispheres and is accompanied by loss of consciousness; in the latter, abnormal activity is limited to part of one cerebral hemisphere only. Generalized seizures usually are characterized by rhythmic, tonic-clonic muscle contractions, or convulsions, although nonconvulsive generalized seizures also occur. Partial seizures can be differentiated further into seizures during which cognition is maintained (simple partial) and seizures during which cognition is impaired (complex partial). The term "cognition" is defined as involving at least two of the five features—perception, attention, emotion, memory, and executive function [36-37]. Partial seizures may become generalized (partial with secondary generalization). Importantly, seizures in children occur as frequently as in adults, however, are more easily inducible by any source, especially in hot environment.

After exposure to NA, the individual would lose consciousness, then immediately will start to convulse and, several minutes later, cease to breath. If no anti-epileptic drug is applied at this stage, the victim is likely to develop irreversible neuronal damage [38,39] within specific brain nuclei. The neurotoxic effects of NA are related to excessive buildup of ACh [40] and overstimulation of central muscarinic receptors. This leads to over-excitation at the cortical or limbic structures, resulting in convulsions and formation of brain lesions typical to this type of intoxication usually located within specific brain nuclei [38]. Pretreatment or early administration of muscarinic receptor antagonists blocks development of the seizure wave and of the structural brain damage is eventually evitable [41]. If untreated, the electro-neural activity recruits other neurotransmitter systems for its propagation (*e.g.*, NMDA receptors); consequently, convulsion may become refractory to muscarinic receptor antagonists.

The role of glutamate receptors in the propagation and maintenance of NA-induced seizures is currently acknowledged, based on the released glutamate in the brain and neuronal death. The NA-induced sustained seizure activity is thought to result in the release of excessive amounts of glutamate, which by itself is directly neurotoxic if present at high concentrations [42]. Moreover, glutamate further stimulates the release of ACh [43], contributing to augment excitatory stimulation and to the prolongation of the seizure. Glutamate apparently plays a major excitotoxic role in NA-induced death. Thus, the sequence of events resulting in brain damage after organophosphates (OP) intoxication may be summarized as follows:

- NA transverses the blood–brain barrier, inhibits brain AChE and leads to an increase in ACh in the CNS
- Excess of ACh triggers seizure activity in susceptible brain areas
- Noncholinergic cross-points are recruited and the entire process of convulsions becomes refractory to muscarinic receptor antagonists
- Seizure-induced neural activation cause the release of excessive amounts of glutamate from stimulated glutamatergic neurons
- The resulting excess of glutamate damages adjacent neurons, leading to death.

Signs and Symptoms

The systemic manifestations of convulsive ictal activity include loss of consciousness, hypertension, tachycardia, tachypnea, and hyperglycemia from sympathetic stimulation. With more prolonged convulsions, skeletal muscle damage, lactic acidosis, and, rarely, frank rhabdomyolysis may ensue [44-45]. Autonomic discharge and bulbar muscle involvement may result in urinary or fecal incontinence, vomiting (with significant aspiration risk), tongue biting, and airway impairment. The classic signs and symptoms of NA poisoning are shown in Table **1**. In addition to the muscarinic and nicotinic synaptic hyperactivity [46-47], the central effects lead to apprehension, dizziness, amnesia, seizures, coma, and respiratory depression [48]. Exposure to lower – although long-term – doses of NAs leads to irritability, fatigue, loss of concentration, and memory loss. Nevertheless, even in the latter conditions, individuals that suffer from chronic illness such as compromised cardio-pulmonary function may suffer from hypoxia, which can rapidly lead to anoxic brain damage, terminating in seizures and cardiovascular collapse, and death.

Treatment

Treatment of seizures, as one of the symptoms of injury, induced by NA intoxicants in case of mass casualty, have several considerations to be made (see detailed reviews elsewhere [34, 49, 50]. They are as follows:

1. Preparedness requires clear hierarchy in the organization

2. Pre-hospital medical and para-medical teams, equipments, and protocol readiness with regard to transportation, decontamination areas, and pre-established decision empowering those who are in charge of delivering administrative and medical orders, the individuals that process the detailed information obtained from the first aid groups to arrive in the scene, and determine the number of contingencies to be sent thereafter, as well as specific Triage rules, if needed.

3. Toxicologists dictating pharmaceutical decisions and that will be in contact with regional/governmental authorities

4. Neurologists or internists whose specialty would be treatment of seizures in the emergency department (ED)

5. Administrative director that will be empowered to allocate victims in various intensive care areas based on their level of consciousness, associated pathologies and responsiveness to treatment

6. In-house medical and administrative preparations (evacuation of regular in-patients, ED and ICU preparedness, equipment distribution, *etc.*)

7. Antidotal drugs must be administered promptly and effectively. Drugs to be used should therefore be pre-made pharmaceuticals, where there is no need to mix compounds at site and no calculations to be made under chaotic pressure. The first aid drugs need to be well recognized deposited in familiar places.

8. Drills must be repeatedly done and all protocols executed smoothly.

Pre-Hospital Assistance

Efficient deployment of hazardous materials (HazMat) teams is critical to control a non-conventional NA attack. Although all major cities and emergency medical systems have plans and equipment in place to address this situation [50], physicians and other health professionals must be aware of principles involved in managing population exposed to these agents. Chemical weapon agents have a high potential for secondary contamination from victims to first-aid responders. This requires that medical treatment facilities clearly define procedures for handling contaminated casualties, some of whom will be transported to the main medical facility. Precautions must be used until thorough decontamination has been performed and the specific chemical agent is identified. Health care professionals must first protect themselves (*e.g.*, by using protective suits, respiratory protection, and chemical-resistant gloves) because secondary contamination with even small amounts of these substances (particularly NAs such as VX) may be lethal [51].

If the released hazard is persistent and transmissible, decontamination is essential outside the medical facility. In some countries, level C–protected medical staff or paramedics can now operate in this area and work alongside with fire personnel in providing (1) triage, based on the patient's medical status; (2) immediate life support measures (TOXALS); (3) immediate antidotal and other pharmacologic support; and (4) decontamination and transfer to medical facility. Noteworthy, do not induce emesis because of the risk of pulmonary aspiration of gastric contents which may result from abrupt respiratory arrest, seizures, or vomiting.

Once the emergency medical staff (EMS) arrives at the location of the event, and after ensuring the safety of the personnel, the most senior medical officer of the EMS should assess the area and call for extra help as required. Any injury to individuals, either blunt trauma or NA, would require patent airway and oxygenation (if no fear of explosion). These are hardly available in the pre-hospital setup in a mass casualty event. If possible (given the chaotic scenario) primary triage proceeds are focused in four directions:

1. Immediate: for those requiring urgent evacuation;

2. Delayed: for casualties that can safely wait for transfer;

3. Expectant: for dying patients who should be provided with supportive treatment only;

4. Deceased: should be positioned in a remote area.

Life Support Measures

Urgent treatment is provided according to the advanced trauma life support (ATLS) guidelines. The ease, by which A-B-C steps could be applicable, such as the ease with which caregivers can move around and exercise resuscitation, is unpredictable due to environmental conditions and physical limitations. Airway protection, the first and most important step toward salvage of an individual presenting with respiratory distress, may be difficult to achieve even by skilled anesthesiologists. Tracheal intubation is very difficult in such scenarios, while a laryngeal mask airway (LMA) can be inserted with comparative ease, even by non-anesthesiologists [52]. The insertion of an LMA would not require the patient to have an intravenous line in place, a procedure that would be very difficult in the field.

Ben-Abraham *et al* demonstrated that an intra-osseous emergency access instead of an intravenous line inserted by physicians wearing full protective gear was easy and rapid, and that its use during emergent treatment of toxic mass casualty could be of potential benefit [53].

The probable unavailability of sufficient numbers of variable automated ventilators, both at the scene and in hospital, and the subsequent need for 1:1 individuals to manually ventilate the injured, poses challenges to the anesthesiologist [34, 54]. These issues relate to the grade of preparedness ahead of time practiced by the local and central authorities.

Drug potency and speed of activity are two factors to be considered when evaluating a potential drug that would protect the injured and would allow for optimal recovery. This is also true for effective anticonvulsant drug. Most previous anticonvulsant studies focused exclusively on seizures elicited by the NA soman. The dose of drug chosen should be sufficient to stop seizures elicited by all agents rapidly and should show efficacy across a wide range of agent exposure levels. Nevertheless, one has to remember that above all, airway protection and maintenance of proper cardiac output are essential to save brain from damage, and to allow effective anticonvulsant activity. In this regard it is recommended not to induce emesis because of the substantial risk of pulmonary aspiration of gastric contents which may result from abrupt respiratory arrest, seizures, or vomiting.

The most immediate concern in the treatment of acute NA poisoning is to establish an airway and provide adequate ventilation and oxygenation, using advance life support techniques including intubation and ventilation with supplemental oxygen. Mouth-to-mouth resuscitation is not recommended because of the high risk for rescuer contamination and poisoning. Note that oropharyngeal intubation may be difficult owing to trismus from muscular spasm and fasciculation's or seizures [55-56]. The initial advanced life support measures are further and extensively detailed elsewhere [34, 57]. Initial ventilation may demonstrate marked airway resistance due to severe bronchial constriction and bronchorrhea. Therefore, atropine should be administered as soon as possible by whatever route is available to reverse the muscarinic effects of the NA. For detailed ventilatory solutions see previous reviews [34, 57].

PHARMACOLOGICAL NA ANTAGONISTS

The early administration of antidotes is critical in the treatment of NA poisoning. Antidotal therapy for NA poisoning includes atropine, an oxime, and a benzodiazepine (BZD). The decision to administer an antidote is based on the severity of poisoning and route of exposure, as well as the head-toxicologist's advice.

Drug potency and speed of activity are two factors to be considered when evaluating a potential drug that would protect the injured and would allow for optimal recovery. This is also true for effective anticonvulsant drug. Most previous anticonvulsant studies focused exclusively on seizures elicited by the NA soman. The dose of drug chosen should be sufficient to stop seizures elicited by all agents rapidly and should show efficacy across a wide range of agent exposure levels. Nevertheless, one has to remember that above all, airway protection and maintenance of proper cardiac output are essential to save brain from damage, and to allow effective anticonvulsant activity.

Pre-hospital drug administration consists of a triade of atropine, oximes and BZD, all aiming at quickly counteracting and possibly reversing NA's neural effects. The problematic port of access has previously been discussed [34]. Intra-osseous access was shown to allow for the administration of drugs and fluids to the dehydrated individuals [53]. Intra-tracheal mode of administration, a frequent clinical way of administrating drugs in patients, appears inapplicable under the given conditions because of the copious amounts of secretions generated by the NA. The adverse effects of atropine and administration protocols are discussed elsewhere [57].

The MARK I kit (atropine, 2 mg, plus 2-pralidoxime chloride, 600 mg) and diazepam, 10 mg, were developed for military use intramuscularly, and are now stockpiled by civilian responders as autoinjectors. In-hospital emergency physicians will probably see patients who had already been treated with them [58] and will continue to use them. Intramuscular dosing saves time during initial treatment by emergency responders and in the treatment of patients in whom rapid gain of intravenous access is difficult. Although diazepam is the most frequently recommended BZD [59], lorazepam and midazolam are also effective in treating seizures from NAs, but barbiturates, phenytoin, and other anticonvulsant medications are not [60] (Table **2**). Phenytoin needs a blood-infused loading dose which excludes its applicability in emergency mass casualty events.

There is no dose limit for the total amount of atropine administered, and the end point of the therapy should be determined by clinical stabilization. Patients who require continued antidotal treatment after the initial improvement should be suspected of having continued dermal NA absorption and undergo repeated decontamination.

Oximes are the second important antidote in the treatment of NA poisoning [61]. Their primary role is to reactivate AChE after it has been phosphorylated by a NA, by removing the NA from its active site, if still feasible. They act at the nicotinic synapse, restoring neuromuscular function and reversing skeletal muscle paralysis. For preventive and therapeutic administration of oximes, including newer compounds, see elsewhere [35, 62].

Noteworthy, in the United States, 2-pralidoxime chloride (2-PAM, pyridine-2-aldoxime methochloride, Protopam) is the only oxime currently approved by the FDA for the treatment of organophosphate or NA poisoning. However, other oximes, including obidoxime, pralidoxime iodide (2-PAM iodide), pralidoxime mesylate (P2S), pralidoxime methylsulfate, and trimedoxime (TMB4), are available in other countries. The differences in the oxime effectiveness are mainly due to the considerable variation in aging rates of the various NAs, the oxime effectiveness, and the animal experimental model, including human used [63-66]. Several countries, including Canada, Sweden, the former Yugoslav confederation, and the Czech Republic, are investigating HI-6 as their oxime of choice for the treatment of NA poisoning.

The addition of BZD has been shown to improve survival from NA poisoning and to decrease the development of permanent brain damage [67-68]. Diazepam is available in an autoinjector and is issued (in addition to 3 Mark I autoinjectors) to U.S. military personnel as part of their NA medical countermeasure kit. It is recommended that a BZD be administered for any type of seizure activity, be it moderate or severe, following NA poisoning, and even before the development of seizures (Table **2**).

BZDs are the only anticonvulsant medications that are proven and authorized in patients with seizures from NAs. Clinically used anticonvulsant drugs administered for status epilepticus would wastes valuable time. Although not FDA-approved for this indication, midazolam is the most efficacious BZD in studies in animals [69]. Potential advances in seizure treatment regard the use of intramuscular and/or intranasal midazolam as the pre-hospital / mass casualty anticonvulsant of choice, and the potential use of ketamine as an adjunct for the treatment of prolonged NA–induced seizures appears in the literature. Nevertheless, anti-convulsive adequate dosing of such drugs may be associated with medium-deep sedative state that would require maintenance of adequate respiratory support.

Nonselective glutamate receptor antagonists, such as felbamate, acting either on *N*-methyl-D-aspartate (NMDA) receptor or on non-NMDA receptors [70], and selective NMDA receptor–channel blockers, such as dizocilpine (MK-801), *N*-[1-(2-thienyl)-cyclohexanyl]- piperidine (TCP), and procyclidine [71-72] are known to serve as potent NA-induced antiepileptic compounds. The latter are even effective if administered when seizure is already fully developed and muscarinic receptor antagonists are ineffective. Among the clinically available compounds, ketamine is a NMDA receptor ion-channel blocker with neuroprotective and anti-epileptic properties [73-74]. Its known psychomimetic side-effects pose limitation to its use. Dextromethorphan and its active metabolite dextrorphan are also NMDA receptor antagonists. Both possess anti-excitotoxic and anti-epileptic properties [75]. Finally, memantine is another promising antagonist of the NMDA receptor, which acts at the phencyclidine binding site. It reduces the degree of convulsions and protects animals from the lethal effects of soman [76]. NMDA receptor antagonists exert anticonvulsant effects against NA-induced seizures when both administered before and after seizures have started [70-71]. This antiepileptic effect is optimal when the drugs are administered concurrently with muscarinic receptor antagonists, blocking the recruitment of glutamate receptors and hence the maintenance of seizure activity and irreversible functional and structural brain damage. If administered without the antimuscarinic, some studies have demonstrated these drugs may exert lethal effects on respiratory function in soman-intoxicated subjects because of their potential to exacerbate the NA-induced the respiratory depressant effects rather than to exert their anti-epileptogenic effects [77].

HYDROGEN CYANIDE

The devastating action of cyanide gas has been dug into the memory of mankind by its inhuman use for the genocide of the Jewish people by the Nazis. It was also used during WWI under the name of Vincennite as warfare agent [78]. Hydrogen cyanide gas has a high vapor pressure and low molecular weight, so that deadly concentrations in the open air are difficult to achieve. Nevertheless, a terrorist attack inside buildings cannot be excluded and could cause many deaths.

Symptoms

The first feeling after cyanide inhalation is cold in the nose and throat followed by a burning sensation with the smell of bitter almonds [79]. Interestingly, only ~50% of the European population is able to smell this typical odor. Headache, a transient CNS stimulation, dizziness and vertigo are the early stage's symptoms of cyanide poisoning.

This is followed by coma, seizures and opisthotonus [80]. Early respiratory arrest with tachycardia changing into bradycardia and cardiac arrest are the most severe and striking symptoms [81]. This occurs within approximately 5 min after severe poisoning. Depending on the ambient concentration of the poison, a certain short period of time may be left for therapeutic effective measures.

Treatment

The diagnosis of cyanide poisoning must be done carefully. The initial treatment should be focused on maintaining the ABCs. Maintaining patient airway and appropriate oxygenation are of utmost priority. Standard antiarrhythmogenic medications are appropriate for the treatment of cyanide-induced arrhythmias. Vasopressors may be required as well.

Any potentially exposed skin or eyes to the toxic agent require prompt decontamination by copious irrigation with saline or water. Currently, a therapeutic mode of known or suspected cyanide intoxication consists of the administration of amyl nitrite, sodium nitrite, and subsequently sodium thiosulfate. Using this combination of medications, at pre-hospital and emergency conditions, amyl nitrite pearls should be broken open and the patient allowed breathing a pearl content for 30 seconds each minute. The pearl is then used up and therefore a new pearl is needed every 3 or 4 minutes. Once intravenous access has been established, 300 mg of sodium nitrite (one 10-mL ampule of 3% solution) for adults, and 0.12–0.33 mL/kg for pediatrics, can be administered for as long as necessary. Because sodium nitrite is a potent vasodilator, hypotension can ensue. Following sodium nitrite administration, sodium thiosulfate should be administered at a dose of 12.5g (one 50-mL ampule of a 25% solution) for adults, and 1.65 mL/kg for pediatrics, IV.

Hydroxocobalamin is an antidote for severe cyanide toxicity. This drug has a cobalt ion, which allows it to chelate the cyanide and form cyanocobalamin (vitamin B12), which is eliminated in the urine [82]. Hydroxocobalamin reduces whole blood cyanide levels and increases urinary cyanide excretion, and it has the added advantage of not causing methemoglobinemia or hypotension [83]. Its efficacy and safety have also been proved in fire victims with cyanide intoxication [84]. In Europe, hydroxocobalamin has been included in antidote kits in many paramedic units and hospital emergency rooms for the treatment of patients who have inhaled smoke during a fire or the victims of a chemical emergency in which cyanide intoxication is suspected.

Hydroxocobalamin is still an investigational drug in the United States; nevertheless, similar measures have been proposed for the United States [85]. Because it acts rapidly and can be administered safely by both emergency responders and hospital clinicians, the development and stockpiling of this medication might improve public health preparedness in the United States [85].

Thiosulfate, a slower-acting agent, may have a synergistic effect when administered after hydroxocobalamin. Cyanocobalamin can give up its cyanide to rhodanese, the enzyme that converts thiosulfate to thiocyanate, regenerating hydroxocobalamin to bind more cyanide in the case of prolonged exposures [86].

SODIUM MONOFLUORO-ACETATE

Sodium monofluoroacetate (SMFA) is both chemically and toxicologically identical to the fluoroacetate found in certain poisonous plants in Australia, South Africa, and South America [87-88]. SMFA is also known as ''1080,'' referring to SMFA's catalog number that became its brand name. SMFA was discovered by German military chemists during World War II [89].

Properties and Routes of Exposure

The synthetic form of the SMFA exists as a white powder (similar in appearance to flour or powdered sugar) that remains stable for long periods of time. It is odorless, tasteless, and readily dissolves in water [87]. When present in natural water sources, it degrades within 7 days because of its metabolism by microorganisms within those environments. In water devoid of microorganisms, SMFA appears to remain stable [90]. It is insoluble in organic solvents such as ethanol or vegetable oils [91]. The only reported distinguishing characteristic is that it has a weak vinegar taste when mixed with water [91]. It is heat stable; it does not decompose until temperatures approach

200°C. SMFA is highly toxic to vertebrates, although the sensitivity of different species varies dramatically. In humans, the estimated lethal poisoning dose (LD_{50}) ranges from 2 to 5 mg/kg body weight [91].

The compound 1080 is well absorbed from the gastrointestinal tract, the respiratory tract, open wounds, mucus membranes, and ocular exposure [87]. Most human exposures reported in the medical literature have been through ingestion. Toxicity has been reported to be the same whether it is administered orally, subcutaneously, intramuscularly, or intravenously [87]. Dusts containing SMFA are effectively toxic by inhalation [87].

Symptoms

Clinical signs and symptoms are nonspecific. There is latency of 30 min to 3 hours following the contact with the compound by any route [88, 92-93]. However, delayed onset of symptoms has been reported up to 20 hours [91]; exposure to massive doses may reduce period of latency. In animal studies, the early stages of poisoning consist of lethargy, vomiting, trembling, excessive salivation, incontinence, muscular weakness, incoordination, hypersensitivity to sensory stimuli, and respiratory distress. Early neurological signs include muscular twitches of the face, such as nystagmus and blepharospasm. These then progress to generalized seizures, initially tonic and then becoming cyclically tonic–clonic with periods of lucidity in between [93]. Partial paralysis may be seen that lasts for prolonged time periods. Death typically results from depression of the respiratory center, cardiovascular failure, and/or ventricular fibrillation [88, 93- 94].

Treatment

There is no specific antidote for SMFA toxicity, and therapy is primarily focused on supportive care. Even though activated charcoal binds SMFA, it does not appear to decrease mortality rates [95]. Because SMFA induces hypocalcemia, calcium supplementation through administration of either calcium gluconate or calcium chloride has been shown to be of benefit [96-97]. In animal models, sodium succinate has been shown to be of benefit as a potential antidote to revive the Krebs cycle [96]. Because of the reported potential for delayed clinical effects, patients who have known oral exposure to SMFA should be observed for a minimum of 24 hours following exposure.

Table 1: Symptoms and Signs of NA Poisoning by Type of Cholinergic Receptor and Target Organ

Receptor	Target Organ	Symptoms and Signs
Muscarinic	Iris muscle; ciliary muscle accommodation	Miosis; spasm of the eyelids; nausea and vomiting; headache
	Conjunctival vessels	Vasodilation and hyperemia
	Nasal glands	Rhinorrhea and hyperemia
	Bronchial glands	Increased secretion
	Bronchial muscles	Bronchoconstriction; tightness in the chest; expiratory wheezing; dyspnea
	Gastrointestinal tract	Anorexia; nausea; vomiting; abdominal cramps; diarrhea; tenesmus; involuntary defecation
	Sweat glands	Increased activity
	Salivary glands	Increased activity
	Lacrimal glands	Lacrimation (not usually marked)
	Heart	Bradycardia; occasionally tachycardia
	Bladder	Frequency; involuntary micturition
Nicotinic	Skeletal muscle	Weakness; fatigue; fasciculations; cramps; flaccid paralysis (early effects on respiratory muscles may produce dyspnea)
	Autonomic ganglia	Pallor; occasional elevation of blood pressure
Muscarinic and nicotinic	Central nervous system	Anxiety; restlessness; headache; depression; memory failure; impaired concentration; slurred speech; depression of respiratory and cardiovascular centers; Cheyne-Stokes respiration; non-responsiveness; flaccidity; hypertonicity; seizures; coma; death

Table 2: Pro and Cons of various pharmacological interventions in seizure events.

Compound	Pro	Con
Diazepam	Familiar to all physicians Available for IM injection FDA approved for NA	Painful on injection Less potent than other BZDs in combating seizures
Midazolam	IV, IM, intranasal*, PR*	Non FDA approved
Lorivan	Oral, IV	Non FDA approved
Sodium Thiopentone	Effective for resistant seizures	Non FDA approved Produced as powder Cardiodepressant Causes bronchospasm IV only
Scopolamine	Familiar to ED and CCM IV, IM	Non FDA approved
Ketamine Dextromethorphan	Familiar to ED and CCM IV, IM, oral* Non cardiodepressants Indirect sympathomimetics	Non FDA approved May exacerbate upper airway secretions

*Consider irrelevant in mass casualty (CMW) scenario

Legend: PR, rectally; CCM, critical care medicine

REFERENCES

[1]   Bajgar J. Complex view on poisoning with nerve agents and organophosphates. Acta Medica (Hradec Kralove) 2005; 48: 3-21.

[2]   Barthold CL, Schier JG. Organic phosphorus compounds--nerve agents. Crit Care Clin 2005; 21: 673-89, v-vi.

[3]   Layish I, Krivoy A, Rotman E, Finkelstein A, Tashma Z, Yehezkelli Y. Pharmacologic prophylaxis against nerve agent poisoning. Isr Med Assoc J 2005; 7: 182-7. Review.

[4]   Schechter G. CNS diseases congress: advances in therapeutics, tools and trials. 28-29 June 2004, Strategic Research Institute, Philadelphia, PA, USA. Expert Rev Neurother. 2004; 4: 747-9.

[5]   Bajgar J, Sevelová L, Krejcová G, et al. Biochemical and behavioral effects of soman vapors in low concentrations. Inhal Toxicol 2004; 16: 497-507.

[6]   Brown MA, Brix KA. Review of health consequences from high-, intermediate- and low-level exposure to organophosphorus nerve agents. J Appl Toxicol 1998; 18: 393-408.

[7]   Joosen MJ, Jousma E, van den Boom TM, et al. Long-term cognitive deficits accompanied by reduced neurogenesis after soman poisoning. Neurotoxicology 2009; 30: 72-80.

[8]   Kassa J, Koupilová M, Vachek J. Long-term effects of low-level sarin inhalation exposure on the spatial memory of rats in a T-maze. Acta Medica (Hradec Kralove) 2001; 44: 93-6.

[9]   McDonough JH Jr, Smith RF, Smith CD. Behavioral correlates of soman-induced neuropathology: deficits in DRL acquisition. Neurobehav Toxicol Teratol 1986; 8: 179-87.

[10] Morita H, Yanagisawa N, Nakajima T, et al. Sarin poisoning in Matsumoto, Japan. Lancet 1995; 346: 290-3.

[11] Myhrer T, Andersen JM, Nguyen NH, Aas P. Soman-induced convulsions in rats terminated with pharmacological agents after 45 min: neuropathology and cognitive performance. Neurotoxicology 2005; 26: 39-48.

[12] Baille V, Clarke PG, Brochier G, et al. Soman-induced convulsions: the neuropathology revisited. Toxicology 2005; 215: 1-24.

[13] Hayward IJ, Wall HG, Jaax NK, Wade JV, Marlow DD, Nold JB. Decreased brain pathology in organophosphate-exposed rhesus monkeys following benzodiazepine therapy. J Neurol Sci 1990; 98: 99-106.

[14] Shih YH, Wu SC. Sorption kinetics of selected volatile organic compounds in human. Environ Toxicol Chem 2002; 21: 2067-74.

[15] Misulis KE, Clinton ME, Dettbarn WD, Gupta RC. Differences in central and peripheral neural actions between soman and diisopropyl fluorophosphate, organophosphorus inhibitors of acetylcholinesterase. Toxicol Appl Pharmacol 1987; 89: 391-8.

[16] Lemercier G, Carpentier P, Sentenac-Roumanou H, Morelis P. Histological and histochemical changes in the central nervous system of the rat poisoned by an irreversible anticholinesterase organophosphorus compound. Acta Neuropathol 1983; 61: 123-9.

[17] McLeod, CG. Pathology of nerve agents: perspectives on medical management. Fundam Appl Toxicol 1985; 5: S10–S16.

[18] McDonough JH Jr, Shih TM. Neuropharmacological mechanisms of nerve agent-induced seizure and neuropathology. Neurosci Biobehav Rev 1997; 21: 559-79.

[19] Cole AE, Nicoll RA. The pharmacology of cholinergic excitatory responses in hippocampal pyramidal cells. Brain Res 1984; 305: 283-90.

[20] Madison DV, Lancaster B, Nicoll RA. Voltage clamp analysis of cholinergic action in the hippocampus. J Neurosci 1987; 7: 733-41.

[21] Washburn MS, Moises HC. Electrophysiological and morphological properties of rat basolateral amygdaloid neurons *in vitro*. J Neurosci 1992; 12: 4066-79.

[22] Womble MD, Moises HC. Muscarinic inhibition of M-current and a potassium leak conductance in neurones of the rat basolateral amygdala. J Physiol 1992; 457: 93-114.

[23] Egorov AV, Unsicker K, von Bohlen und Halbach O. Muscarinic control of graded persistent activity in lateral amygdala neurons. Eur J Neurosci 2006; 24: 3183-94.

[24] Yajeya J, De La Fuente A, Criado JM, Bajo V, Sánchez-Riolobos A, Heredia M. Muscarinic agonist carbachol depresses excitatory synaptic transmission in the rat basolateral amygdala *in vitro*. Synapse 2000; 38: 151-60.

[25] Fernández de Sevilla D, Buño W. Presynaptic inhibition of Schaffer collateral synapses by stimulation of hippocampal cholinergic afferent fibres. Eur J Neurosci 2003; 17: 555-8.

[26] Fukudome Y, Ohno-Shosaku T, Matsui M, *et al.* Two distinct classes of muscarinic action on hippocampal inhibitory synapses: M2-mediated direct suppression and M1/M3-mediated indirect suppression through endocannabinoid signalling. Eur J Neurosci 2004; 19: 2682-92.

[27] Salgado H, Bellay T, Nichols JA, *et al.* Muscarinic M2 and M1 receptors reduce GABA release by Ca2+ channel modulation through activation of PI3K/Ca2+ -independent and PLC/Ca2+ -dependent PKC. J Neurophysiol 2007; 98: 952-65.

[28] Lallement G, Carpentier P, Collet A, Pernot-Marino I, Baubichon D, Blanchet G. Effects of soman-induced seizures on different extracellular amino acid levels and on glutamate uptake in rat hippocampus. Brain Res 1991; 563: 234-40.

[29] Wade JV, Samson FE, Nelson SR, Pazdernik TL. Changes in extracellular amino acids during soman- and kainic acid-induced seizures. J Neurochem 1987; 49: 645-50.

[30] Grasshoff C, Gillessen T, Thiermann H, Wagner E, Szinicz L. The effect of acetylcholinesterase-inhibition on depolarization-induced GABA release from rat striatal slices. Toxicology 2003; 184: 149-56.

[31] Solberg Y, Belkin M. The role of excitotoxicity in organophosphorous nerve agents central poisoning. Trends Pharmacol Sci 1997; 18: 183-5.

[32] Lallement G, Clarençon D, Masqueliez C, *et al.* Nerve agent poisoning in primates: antilethal, anti-epileptic and neuroprotective effects of GK-11. Arch Toxicol 1998; 72: 84-92.

[33] Shih TM, McDonough JH Jr. Organophosphorus nerve agents-induced seizures and efficacy of atropine sulfate as anticonvulsant treatment. Pharmacol Biochem Behav 1999; 64: 147-53.

[34] Ben Abraham R, Rudick V, Weinbroum AA. Practical Guidelines for Acute Care of Victims of Bioterrorism: Conventional Injuries and Concomitant Nerve Agent Intoxication. Anesthesiology 2002; 97: 989–1004.

[35] Weinbroum AA. Pathophysiological and clinical aspects of combat anticholinesterase poisoning. Br Med Bul 2005; 72: 119–33.

[36] Blume WT, Lüders HO, Mizrahi E, Tassinari C, van Emde Boas W, Engel J Jr. Glossary of descriptive terminology for ictal semiology: Report of the ILAE task force on classification and terminology. Epilepsia 2001; 42: 1212-8.

[37] Engel J Jr. Progress in epilepsy: reducing the treatment gap and the promise of biomarkers. Curr Opin Neurol 2008; 21: 150-4.

[38] McDonough JH Jr, McLeod CG Jr, Nipwoda MT. Direct microinjection of soman or VX into the amygdala produces repetitive limbic convulsions and neuropathology. Brain Res 1987; 435: 123-37.

[39] Churchill L, Pazdernik TL, Jackson JL, *et al.* Soman-induced brain lesions demonstrated by muscarinic receptor autoradiography. Neurotoxicology 1985; 6: 81-90.

[40] Lallement G, Carpentier P, Collet A, Baubichon D, Pernot-Marino I, Blanchet G. Extracellular acetylcholine changes in rat limbic structures during soman-induced seizures. Neurotoxicology 1992; 13: 557-67.

[41] McDonough JH Jr, Jaax NK, Crowley RA, Mays MZ, Modrow HE. Atropine and/or diazepam therapy protects against soman-induced neural and cardiac pathology. Fundam Appl Toxicol 1989; 13: 256-76.

[42]   Faden AI, Salzman S. Pharmacological strategies in CNS trauma. Trends Pharmacol Sci 1992; 13: 29-35.

[43]   Anderson JJ, Kuo S, Chase TN. Endogenous excitatory amino acids tonically stimulate striatal acetylcholine release through NMDA but not AMPA receptors. Neurosci Lett 1994; 176: 264-8.

[44]   Engel J, Pedley TA, Aicardi J, Dichter MA. Epilepsy: Causes and Consequences. In: Hauser WA, Hesdorffer DC, Eds. New York: Demos; 1990.

[45]   Orringer CE, Eustace JC, Wunsch CD, Gardner LB. Natural history of lactic acidosis after grand-mal seizures: A model for the study of an anion-gap acidosis not associated with hyperkalemia. N Engl J Med 1977; 297: 796-9.

[46]   Amitai Y, Almog S, Singer R, Hammer R, Bentur Y, Danon YL. Atropine poisoning in children during the Persian Gulf crisis. A national survey in Israel. JAMA 1992; 268: 630-2.

[47]   Kozer E, Mordel A, Haim SB, Bulkowstein M, Berkovitch M, Bentur Y. Pediatric poisoning from trimedoxime (TMB4) and atropine automatic injectors. J Pediatr 2005; 146: 41-4.

[48]   Romig LE. Pediatric triage: a system to JumpSTART your triage of young patients at MCIs. JEMS 2002; 27: 52-58.

[49]   Drummond GB. Controlling the airway: skill and science. Anesthesiology 2002; 97: 771-3.

[50]   Murray MJ, Merridew CG. Anesthesiologists Now Must Prepare for Biologic, Nuclear, or Chemical Terrorism. Apsf Newsletter 2002; 17: 1-20.

[51]   Weinbroum AA, Rudick V, Paret G, Kluger Y, Ben Abraham R. Anaesthesia and critical care considerations in nerve agent warfare trauma casualties. Resuscitation 2000; 47: 113-23.

[52]   Flaishon R, Sotman A, Friedman A, Ben-Abraham R, Rudick V, Weinbroum AA. Laryngeal mask airway insertion by anesthetists and nonanesthetists wearing unconventional protective gear: a prospective, randomized, crossover study in humans. Anesthesiology 2004; 100: 267-73.

[53]   Ben-Abraham R, Gur I, Vater Y, Weinbroum AA. Intraosseous emergency access by physicians wearing full protective gear. Acad Emerg Med 2003; 10: 1407-10.

[54]   Ben-Abraham R, Gur I, Bar-Yishay E, *et al*. Application of a cuirass and institution of biphasic extra-thoracic ventilation by gear-protected physicians. J Crit Care 2004; 19: 36-41.

[55]   Blank IH, Griesemer RD, Gould E. The penetration of an anticholinesterase agent (sarin) into skin. I. Rate of penetration into excised human skin. J Invest Dermatol 1957; 29: 299-309.

[56]   Sidell F. Sarin and soman: observations on accidental exposures. Edgewood Arsenal Technical Report 4747, DTIC AD769737. Fort Belvoir, VA, Defense Technical Information Center, 1973.

[57]   Dichtwald S, Weinbroum AA. Bioterrorism and the anaesthesiologist's perspective. Best Prac Res Clin Anaesthesiol 2008; 22: 477–502.

[58]   Kales SN, Christiani DC. Acute chemical emergencies. N Engl J Med 2004; 350: 800-8.

[59]   No authors listed. Prevention and treatment of injury from chemical warfare agents. Med Lett Drugs Ther 2002; 44: 1-4.

[60]   Nerve agents. In: Managing hazardous material incidents (MHMI). Vol. 3. Medical management guidelines (MMGs) Atlanta: Agency for Toxic Substances and Disease Registry, 2001.

[61]   Grob D, Johns RJ. Use of oximes in the treatment of intoxication by anticholinesterase compounds in patients with myasthenia gravis. Am J Med 1958; 24: 512-518.

[62]   Worek F, Szinicz L. Atropine and oxime treatment in lethal soman poisoning of anaesthetized guinea-pigs: Hl 7 dimethanesulfide versus HI 6 dichloride. Pharmacol Toxicol 1993; 72: 13–21.

[63]   Dawson RM. Review of oximes available for treatment of nerve agent poisoning. J Appl Toxicol 1994; 14: 317-31.

[64]   Lundy PM, Hansen AS, Hand BT, Boulet CA. Comparison of several oximes against poisoning by soman, tabun and GF. Toxicology 1992; 72: 99-105.

[65]   Worek F, Kirchner T, Backer M, Szinicz L. Reactivation by various oximes of human erythrocyte acetylcholinesterase inhibited by different organophosphorus compounds. Arch Toxicol 1996; 70: 497-503.

[66]   Worek F, Widmann R, Knopff O, Szinicz L. Reactivating potency of obidoxime, pralidoxime, HI 6 and HLo 7 in human erythrocyte acetylcholinesterase inhibited by highly toxic organophosphorus compounds. Arch Toxicol 1998; 72: 237-43.

[67]   Rump S, Kowaczyk M. Management of convulsions in nerve agent acute poisoning: a Polish perspective. J Med Chem Def 2003; 1: 1-14.

[68]   Martin LJ, Doebler JA, Shih TM, Anthony A. Protective effect of diazepam pretreatment on soman-induced brain lesion formation. Brain Res 1985; 325: 287-9.

[69]   McDonough JH Jr, McMonagle J, Copeland T, Zoeffel D, Shih T-M. Comparative evaluation of benzodiazepines for control of soman-induced seizures. Arch Toxicol 1999; 73: 473-8.

[70]   Choi DW. Glutamate neurotoxicity and diseases of the nervous system. Neuron. 1988; 1: 623-34. Review.

[71]   Shih TM. Anticonvulsant effects of diazepam and MK-801 in soman poisoning. Epilepsy Res 1990; 7: 105-16.

[72]   Sparenborg S, Brennecke LH, Jaax NK, Braitman DJ. Dizocilpine (MK-801) arrests status epilepticus and prevents brain damage induced by soman. Neuropharmacology 1992; 31:357-68. Erratum in: Neuropharmacology 1993; 32: 313.

[73] Olney JW, Price MT, Samson L, Labruyere J. The role of specific ions in glutamate neurotoxicity. Neurosci Lett 1986; 65: 65-71.

[74] Croucher MJ, Collins JF, Meldrum BS. Anticonvulsant action of excitatory amino acid antagonists. Science 1982; 216: 899-901.

[75] Choi DW. Dextrorphan and dextromethorphan attenuate glutamate neurotoxicity. Brain Res 1987; 403: 333-6.

[76] Deshpande SS, Smith CD, Filbert MG. Assessment of primary neuronal culture as a model for soman-induced neurotoxicity and effectiveness of memantine as a neuroprotective drug. Arch Toxicol 1995; 69: 384-90.

[77] Rickett DI, Glenn JF, Beers ET. Central respiratory effects versus neuromuscular actions of nerve agents. Neurotoxicology 1986; 7: 225-36.

[78] Paulet G. Hydrocyanic attacks and chemical warfare. Rev Corps Sante Armees Terre Mer Air 1962; 3: 971-93.

[79] Vogel SN, Sultan TR, Ten Eyck RP. Cyanide poisoning. Clin Toxicol 1981; 18: 367-83.

[80] Hall AH, Rumack BH. Clinical toxicology of cyanide. Ann Emerg Med 1986; 15: 1067-74.

[81] Stewart R. Cyanide poisoning. Clin Toxicol 1974; 7:561-4.

[82] Duenas Laita A, Nogué Xarau S. Intoxicacition por el humo de los incendios: tratamiento antidótico a base de vitaminas. Med Clin [Barc] 2000; 114: 658-60.

[83] Forsyth JC, Mueller PD, Becker CE, *et al.* Hydroxocobalamin as a cyanide antidote: safety, efficacy and pharmacokinetics in heavily smoking normal volunteers. J Toxicol Clin Toxicol 1993; 31: 277-94.

[84] Baud FJ, Barriot P, Toffis V, *et al.* Elevated blood cyanide concentrations in victims of smoke inhalation. N Engl J Med 1991; 325: 1761-6.

[85] Sauer SW, Keim ME. Hydroxocobalamin: improved public health readiness for cyanide disasters. Ann Emerg Med 2001; 37: 635-41.

[86] Aaron CK. Cyanide antidotes. In: Goldfrank LR, Flomenbaum NE, Lewin NA, Weisman RS, Howland MA, Hoffman RS, Eds. Goldfrank's toxicologic emergencies. 6th ed. Stamford, Conn.: Appleton & Lange, 1998: 1583-5.

[87] Egekeze JO, Oehme FW. Sodium monofluoroacetate (SMFA, compound 1080): a literature review. Vet Hum Toxicol 1979; 21: 411–6.

[88] Eason C. Sodium monofluoroacetate (1080) risk assessment and risk communication. Toxicology 2002; 181–182: 523–30.

[89] Abraham K. Defazio bill bans poison. The Eugene Weekly. January 12, 2006. Available at: http://www.predatordefense.org/EugeneWeekly.pdf.

[90] Booth LH, Ogilvie SC, Wright GR, Eason CT. Degradation of sodium monofluoroacetate (1080) and fluorocitrate in water. Bull Environ Contam Toxicol 1999; 62: 34–9.

[91] Robinson RF, Griffith JR, Wolowich WR, Nahata MC. Intoxication with sodium monofluoroacetate (compound 1080). Vet Hum Toxicol 2002; 44: 93–5.

[92] Sherley M. The traditional categories of fluoroacetate poisoning signs and symptoms belie substantial underlying similarities. Toxicol Lett 2004; 151: 399–406.

[93] Trabes J, Rason N, Avrahami E. Computed tomography demonstration of brain damage due to acute sodium monofluoroacetate poisoning. J Toxicol Clin Toxicol 1983; 20: 85–92.

[94] Ando J, Shiozu K, Kawasaki H. A selective blockade of the cardiac inotropic effect of adrenaline by sodium monofluoroacetate. Bull Osaka Med Sch 1966; 12: 1–4.

[95] Norris WR, Temple WA, Eason CT, Wright GR, Ataria J, Wickstrom ML. Sorption of fluoroacetate (compound 1080) by Colestipol, activated charcoal and anion-exchange in resins *in vitro* and gastrointestinal decontamination in rats. Vet Hum Toxicol 2000; 42: 269–75.

[96] Omara F, Sisodia CS. Evaluation of potential antidotes for sodium fluoroacetate in mice. Vet Hum Toxicol 1990; 32: 427–31.

[97] Taitelman U, Roy A, Raikhlin-Eisenkraft B, Hoffer E. The effect of monoacetin and calcium chloride on acid-base balance and survival in experimental sodium fluoroacetate poisoning. Arch Toxicol Suppl 1983; 6: 222–7.

CHAPTER 3

Seizures and Other Neurological Symptoms Induced by Organophosphates, Including Warfare Nerve Agents

Adam-Scott Feiner, Bertrand Yersin*, Andreas Stettbacher, Sergei Bankoul, Christophe Baumberger and Pierre-Nicolas Carron

Emergency Service, University Hospital (CHUV), Lausanne, 1011 Switzerland; Swiss Armed Forces, Office of the Surgeon in Chief, Ittigen, 3063 Switzerland, and Swiss Armed Forces, NBC Centre of Competence, Spiez, 3700 Switzerland

Abstract. Acute organophosphate (OP) intoxication is associated with many symptoms and clinical signs, including potentially life-threatening seizures and status epilepticus. Instead of being linked to the direct cholinergic toxidrome, OP-related seizures are more probably linked to the interaction of OPs with acetylcholine-independent neuromodulation pathways, such as GABA and NMDA. The importance of preventing, or recognizing and treating OP-related seizures lies in that, the central nervous system (CNS) damage from OP poisoning is thought to be due to the excitotoxicity of the seizure activity itself rather than a direct toxic effect. Muscular weakness and paralysis occurring 1-4 days after the resolution of an acute cholinergic toxidrome, the intermediate syndrome is usually not diagnosed until significant respiratory insufficiency has occurred; it is nevertheless a major cause of OP-induced morbidity and mortality and requires aggressive supportive treatment. The condition usually resolves spontaneously in 1-2 weeks.

Treatment of OP intoxication relies on prompt diagnosis, and specific and immediate treatment of the life-threatening symptoms. Since patients suffering from OP poisoning can secondarily expose care providers *via* contaminated skin, clothing, hair, or body fluids. EMS and hospital caregivers should be prepared to protect themselves with appropriate protective equipment, isolate such patients, and decontaminate them. After prompt decontamination, the initial priority of patient management is an immediate ABCDE (A : airway, B : breathing, C : circulation, D : dysfunction or disability of the central nervous system, and E : exposure) resuscitation approach, including aggressive respiratory support, since respiratory failure is the usual ultimate cause of death. The subsequent priority is initiating atropine therapy to oppose the muscarinic symptoms and diazepam to prevent or control seizures, with oximes added to enhance acetylcholinesterase (AChE) activity recovery. Large doses of atropine and oximes may be necessary for poisoning due to suicidal ingestions of OP pesticides.

INTRODUCTION

Cholinesterase inhibitors are numerous and include organophosphates, such as warfare nerve agents, and carbamates. For obvious reasons, linked to the dramatic threat they represent for human health and challenges to medical treatment, this chapter will mainly focus on the organophosphate compounds (OP[1]) and their effects on the human nervous system.

Since their discovery by Schrader in Germany during the Second World War, initially studied as insecticides, and then immediately considered as potential warfare agents, more than thirty chemical products have been then synthesized to date, either as warfare nerve agents, herbicides, fungicides, but mainly as pesticides [1].

Despite their common effect of inhibiting acetylcholinesterase (AChE), and thus blocking the normal breakdown of the neurotransmitter acetylcholine, these chemicals produce a large variety of clinical toxic effects in exposed subjects. This variety of clinical problems is explained not only by differences in their physical properties and pharmacokinetics, but also because of their different pharmacological properties, such as for example the specific toxic effects they can have on muscarinic or nicotinic receptors, as well as on other target enzymes, the route of

---

*Address correspondence to Prof Bertrand Yersin: Emergency Service, University Hospital (CHUV), BH 06-429, Lausanne, 1011 Switzerland; Tel +41 21 314 38 74; E-mail: Bertrand.Yersin@chuv.ch

---

[1] Organophosphates will be systematically abbreviated as OPs in all pages of this chapter.

Feng Ru Tang and Weng Keong Loke (Eds)

intoxication (inhalation, ingestion or dermal exposure) or the characteristics of the exposed subject. However the clinical findings may be summarized in four different syndromes: a. the acute cholinergic toxidrome linked to accumulation of acetylcholine at neuromuscular junctions and synapses effecting the CNS, skeletal and smooth muscles as well as exocrine glands, b. the intermediate syndrome characterized by a delayed neuromuscular dysfunction in the days following a significant acute cholinergic toxidrome, c. the organophosphate-induced delayed neuropathy (OPIDN), characterized by a one to five week-delayed neuropathy of unknown cause, and d. the organophosphate-induced chronic neurotoxicity (OPICN), characterized by chronic neuropsychiatric symptoms and signs that last for weeks to years after acute exposure.

Due to their potent insecticide effects, OPs are largely produced, distributed, stockpiled and used, sometimes to excess, all over the world. Accidental exposures, as well as intentional intoxications (suicide attempts) are thus very common. It is estimated that more than three millions OP intoxications occur world-wide, causing more than 200'000 deaths, each year [2]. In particular, Oral ingestion of OP with suicidal intent is particularly frequent in African and Asian developing and emergent countries [2-5]. In addition to these threatening civilian health concerns, the production and accumulation of warfare OP nerve agents by numerous national armies, as well as their recent use by the Iraqis in Kurdistan and the Aum religious group in two consecutive terrorist attacks in Tokyo, have motivated hospital preparedness all over the world, as well as tremendous public health and security efforts in preventing such individual or collective intoxications. It is also to be emphasized that basic and clinical research dealing with understanding the fundamental pathophysiology of OP intoxication and its treatment have to be developed and supported, as the level of evidence we have on these matters is particularly low.

The purpose of this chapter is to review the current information pertaining to the clinical aspects and management of OP intoxication-induced seizures and other neurological symptoms. After reviewing the mechanisms of nervous system toxicity and their clinical presentation, the ways to manage and treat these problems will be summarized.

MECHANISMS OF TOXICITY

The organophosphate (OP) nerve agents and pesticides are heterogeneous substances sharing similar mechanisms of toxicity and potential high mortality in case of acute intoxication. Their reactivity depends on their chemical structures. They act primarily by inhibiting numerous esterase enzymes, but the key factor of OP multi-system toxicity is the irreversible inhibition of the tissue acetylcholinesterase (AChE), both in the central and the peripheral nervous system.

The inactivation of AChE by organophosphates is a multiple-step process. The OP inhibits the AChE enzyme by phosphorylating the serine hydroxyl group at the AChE enzyme's active site. The inhibited enzyme is unable to inactivate acetylcholine, leading to increased levels of acetylcholine at nerve synapses. The accumulation of acetylcholine induces over-stimulation of acetylcholine receptors in synapses of the autonomic nervous system, central nervous system and neuromuscular junction. AChE may be subsequently regenerated by a hydroxyl ion attacking the phosphorylated serine residue (spontaneous reactivation), but this process is much slower than inhibition. In the inactive state, the AChE-OP complex is then prone to "ageing", a process that implies a non-enzymatic hydrolysis of one of the remaining alkyl substituents of the phosphorous moiety, leaving a hydroxyl group in its place. This process of ageing results in irreversible inactivation of AChE, which cannot spontaneously regenerate or be reactivated by oxime antidotes. The time for ageing depends on the nerve agent, the persistence and the concentration of OP. Ageing with soman occurs so fast (some minutes) that no clinically relevant spontaneous reactivation of AChE can occur before ageing has taken place. Hence, the restoration of AChE function depends solely on the relatively slow re-synthesis of new AChE enzymes (the half-life of AChE re-synthesis in the nervous system is about 5 to 7 days). For OP insecticides, ageing is rarely clinically relevant because these agents age at slower rates. In the context of pesticide poisoning, the presence of two methyl groups attached to the phosphorous atom (dimethyl organophosphates) enhances the process of ageing (as opposed to diethyl organophosphates) [6]. Metabolic transformation of OP through oxidative reactions can create active metabolites, some with increased toxicity. Some pesticides or herbicides owe their selectivity to activation by enzymes specific to the target species (7). OP is detoxified by carboxylesterases (soman, sarin, tabun), phosphorylphosphatases (soman, sarin) and the glutathione redox system. The CYP1A2*1F polymorphism is associated with an increase risk of neurological toxicity; cytochrome induction may represent a distinct risk factor [7- 8].

CLINICAL PRESENTATION OF OP INTOXICATION

The Acute Cholinergic Toxidrome

The acute cholinergic crisis develops within a few minutes to several hours after exposure. The severity, timing and symptoms of OP poisoning depend on the substance, dose, route of exposure (inhalation, ingestion, or skin exposure) and duration of exposure (Table **1**) [9]. The cholinergic symptoms are predominantly related to peripheral nicotinic and muscarinic intoxication and occur in the order that the toxin encounters the involved cholinergic synapses (Table **2**) [10-11]. Ingestion of OP nerve agents is rare, but is of major concern for OP pesticide intoxication [1]). In most cases, death occurs during the acute cholinergic phase, from cardiac arrest, respiratory distress or brain toxicity. Direct cardiac toxicity and heart failure have been described in animal studies and case series [13].

Table 1: Nerve gas OPs agent's toxicity [9]

	Soman (GD)	Sarin (GB)	Tabun (GA)	VX
LD 50 (mg/kg)	-	28 mg/kg (skin)	-	-
LCLo (mg/m3)	70 mg/m3	-	150 mg/m3	-
LDLo (mg/kg)	18 mg/m3 (skin) 70 mg/m3 (inhal)	0.03 mg/kg (im)	23 mg/kg (skin) 0.014 mg/kg (iv)	0.086 mg/kg (skin)
TDLo (mg/kg)	-	0.002 mg/kg	-	0.003 mg/kg (im) 0.004 mg/kg (oral)

LD 50 = Lethal Dose 50, the calculated dose that causes death in 50% of individuals

LCLo = Lethal Concentration Low, the lowest concentration of a substance in air that cause death,

LDLo = Lethal Dose Low, the lowest dose of a chemical which tests have shown will be lethal.

TDLo = Toxic Dose Low, the lowest dosage per unit of bodyweight (typically stated in milligrams per kilogram) of a substance known to have produced signs of toxicity.

iv: intravenous

im: intramuscular

inhal: inhalation

Table 2: Symptoms and signs of acute organophosphates poisoning

Overstimulation of the muscarinic receptors in the parasympathetic system	Overstimulation of the nicotinic receptors in the sympathetic system	Overstimulation of the nicotinic and muscarinic receptors in the central nervous system	Overstimulation of the nicotinic receptors of the neuromuscular junction
Diarrhoea, emesis	Tachycardia, hypertension (initially)	Seizures	Weakness
Urination	Sweating	Altered level of consciousness, confusion, coma	Fasciculation followed by flaccid paralysis
Miosis	Mydriasis	Respiratory depression	
Bradycardia, hypotension (later)			
Bronchospasm, bronchorrhea			
Salivation, secretion, rhinorrhea, lacrimation			

Vapour exposure is the most likely contact route in battlefield and in terrorist attacks. The most exposed, and thus first affected synapses are in the pupillary muscle, producing miosis, eye pain and blurred vision. Indeed, in the Tokyo sarin attack, the most common complaint was visual impairment, described by victims as *"the world going black"* [14-15]. The next sites involved are the mouth, nose, pharynx and pulmonary tracts, where cholinergic over-stimulation causes increased secretions and induces bronchospasm. The OP then cross the pulmonary alveolar-capillary membrane and enter the bloodstream, reaching the gastrointestinal tract, resulting in vomiting, diarrhea and abdominal pain. After the gastro-intestinal tract, OP affects the heart, the muscles and the brain. They cause cardiac dysrhythmias, cardiac arrest, hypertension or hypotension, diaphragm dysfunction, and fasciculations. If the motor end-plate hyperstimulation is of sufficient duration, flaccid paralysis will ensue [16].

After dermal contact, the OP will cause localized sweating and fasciculations. The effects may be delayed up to 18 hours. After entering the circulation, OP cause gastrointestinal, respiratory, cardiac and central neurological symptoms. The time course will be much longer than with vapor inhalation and miosis is not always observed. The presence of wounds or cutaneous lesions increases the diffusion rate.

The Intermediate Syndrome

Patients can develop peripheral respiratory failure, after recovering from the cholinergic crisis. This intermediate syndrome is characterized by regression of the acute cholinergic syndrome, and worsening of nicotinic-related symptoms, 24 – 96 hours after exposure. [17]. Physical examination reveals proximal limb paralysis, decreased deep tendon reflex, weakness of respiratory muscles and motor cranial nerve involvement (facial muscle weakness, ptosis)[18]. Diaphragmatic paralysis may lead to respiratory insufficiency. The pathophysiology underlying the intermediate syndrome remains unclear. Pre- and post-synaptic impairment of neuromuscular transmission, with down-regulation of post-synaptic ACh receptors were suggested [18-19]. Inadequate or delayed oxime therapy and exposure to specific OP may also play a role.

With appropriate supportive therapy, recovery occurs 5 – 20 days after the onset of weakness.

The Organophosphate-Induced Delayed Neuropathy (OPIDN)

OP may induce a delayed motor-sensory polyneuropathy within 1- 3 weeks after acute exposure to nerve gases or certain insecticides. OP-induced polyneuropathy is characterized by progressive symmetrical distal axonopathy, beginning 8–14 days after intoxication [20]. The patients present with ascending motor and sensory dysfunction, predominantly in the lower limbs (paresthesia, cramps, pain, diminished or abolished osteo-tendineous reflexes). This neuropathy evolves slowly over several months and is usually self-resolving, with occasional persistence of sensory-motor sequelae. Suspected mechanisms involve the inhibition of neuropathy target esterase (NTE), causing axonal degeneration. This axonal degeneration is characterized by the activation of calcium activated neutral protease (CANP) due to an excessive intake of calcium by the cell [21]. Activation of Ca/calmodulin kinase II is may be responsible for this increased axonal calcium [22].

The Organophosphate-Induced Chronic Neurotoxicity (OPICN)

Chronic intoxication induced by a long-term low-level exposure of OP may induce neuropsychiatric disorders, such as anxiety, insomnia and depression. These physical symptoms are less well-defined and some of the psychiatric symptoms may be related to the post-traumatic stress reaction, rather than to direct chronic toxicity [15, 23].

The Central Neurological Effects of OP Intoxication

The toxicity of OP on the central nervous system is a major factor of morbidity and mortality, and creates a problem for medical management of exposed subjects.

Muscarinic and nicotinic cholinergic receptors are distributed throughout the central nervous system, predominantly within the reticular activating system, basal ganglia, limbic system, cortical and cerebellar projections. Because of the widespread presence of these receptors, OP poisoning can produce a large variety of neurological symptoms. Headaches, vertigo and paresthesia may occur. Centrally mediated respiratory failure, loss of consciousness and convulsions may lead to death within minutes.

Brain damage by OP nerve agents' exposure is primarily due to seizure activity, which can rapidly progress to status epilepticus. The first phase of seizures is induced by increased cholinergic activity in the brain, particularly at muscarinic (M1) sites. The cholinergic activation results in blockade of various potassium channels and activation of calcium-sensitive cation channels on post-synaptic sites. The onset of this first phase appears to be dose-dependent. This cholinergic phase lasts from the time of exposure to several minutes after the onset of the seizures [24].

A second phase of prolonged seizures occurs after minutes, due to increased excitatory amino-acid neurotransmitter release, particularly glutamate and aspartate, and antagonism of the GABA-mediated system. Over-activation of glutamate receptors, including the N-methyl-D-aspartate (NMDA) receptors is of particular importance in seizure and status epilepticus development. Because of the flaccid paralysis caused by prolonged over-stimulation of the nicotinic receptors at the neuromuscular junction, the signs of status epilepticus induced by OP may become subtle or even absent. In such cases, the EEG may be the only method of establishing the diagnosis. In particular, wavelet analysis frequently reveals strong activation in the delta band [25].

Neuronal injuries, permanent brain dysfunction and death may occur after twenty minutes and are strongly correlated with OP-induced seizure. The occurrence, duration and intensity of seizures activity are related to the incidence and severity of brain damage. The increase in delta activity is a possible marker of brain damage. This brain damage is probably due to the high level of extracellular glutamate, elevated intra-neuronal calcium concentration and associated hypoxia. It is hypothesized that status epilepticus-induced NMDA receptor activation leads to increased production of reactive oxygen species (free radicals), nitric oxide (NO) and zinc ions, which mediate the oxidative damage and neuronal loss [1, 26]. In animal studies, brain lesions varied from little or no pathology to extensive brain damage, with infiltration of inflammatory cells [27-28]. The large variability of lesion patterns may be explained by variations in antioxidants capacities or cytochrome heterogeneity between species and individuals.

The hippocampal region (particularly the hippocampus CA1), the amygdala, the piriform cortex and the entorhinal cortex are particularly prone to epileptiform activity and excitotoxic damage after OP intoxication [29]. *In vitro*, animal experiments with electrophysiological and histopathological studies confirm the high sensitivity of the hippocampus and the amygdala, in particular the basolateral nucleus of the amygdale [30-31]. This propensity may be explained by the high expression of the kainate subtype (GluR5KRs) of glutamate receptors [32].The most susceptible brain areas vary between species. Seizures are more frequent in pediatric relative to adult OP poisoning.

Patients surviving an OP' intoxication are at risk of developing a variety of sequellae, with irritability, personality changes, psychotic episodes, deficits in memory and attention, sleep disturbances and non specific neurobehavioral symptoms. Non-lethal soman exposure may also lead to irreversible brain damage [33]. In a cohort study from Sri Lanka, the Glasgow Coma Scale on admission was an effective clinical tool for predicting outcome and death [34].

DIAGNOSIS

The diagnosis of organophosphate compound intoxication can be based on history, such as in the case of voluntary self-harm where the patient admits intake of the toxicant or when an unconscious patient is found with labeled containers; history of chronic or acute occupational exposure (agriculture, flame-retardants); therapeutic application (lice control), recreational use (pet-care products), non-professional environmental exposure, or acts of war and terrorist activity. Clinical signs that point towards OP intoxication include a pungent, garlic odor, confusion, convulsions, coma, or any of the symptoms of muscarinic or nicotinic receptor hyperactivity. Paraclinical work-up can reveal decreased serum or Red Blood Cell AChE activity, although *caveats* maintain due to the interindividual variability of baseline levels; serial measurements demonstrating progressive increase of AChE activity are considered to be diagnostic of AChE–inhibitor exposure [35]. In the immediate post-exposure phase (ca. 24 h post exposure), lymphocyte NTE activity inhibition correlates with the later development of OPIDN (ca 2-3 weeks post exposure), and is indicative of exposure.

The determination of the exact substance involved, beyond a generic identification, is relevant, as OP is an extremely large group of different compounds. They exert a broad spectrum of toxic effects; the presence and/or magnitude of the cholinergic, muscarinic and CNS symptoms (including convulsions) are compound-dependant, as are the subsequent appearance of an intermediate syndrome and OPIDN. Some OPs not only are unable to cause

OPIDN, but in fact are protective when administered prophylacticaly. In addition, as discussed later, the specific oxime antidotes are not equally efficacious towards all OPs. However, the specific toxicological and biochemical assays required for toxicant identification are time-consuming and frequently unavailable, making history and clinical suspicion of paramount importance.

TREATMENT

Initial Management and Decontamination

Initial management of a patient intoxicated by OP is similar to the treatment of any intoxication, and consists first of patient decontamination and care-provider protection. Separating the victim from the source of further intoxication and prevention of healthcare provider and/or equipment contamination are necessary to allow patient care to continue.

Removal of all clothes, washing with copious amounts of warm water (with a mild soap, if available), must take precedence over any other therapeutic maneuver except basic airway clearing (typically head-tilt and jaw-thrust, if feasible & required) and gross control of massive hemorrhage (s.a. with a tourniquet or a compressive bandage).

After decontamination has been completed, and as far as protection of the care providers is insured, an ABCDE resuscitation approach of the patient is mandatory in case of a life-threatening situation. *Airway* control and *Breathing* support (oxygenation and intubation) are of particular importance, as OP intoxication may kill the patient within minutes, due to airway obstruction with secretions and acute respiratory insufficiency due to bronchospasm and respiratory muscle paralysis. *Circulation* management includes immediate intravenous access; cardiac therapies may be necessary in case of dysrythmias (bradycardia or tachycardia), followed by neurological *Disability* assessment and management. *Exposure* as related to decontamination is of course essential; however, if skin decontamination is mandatory, digestive decontamination with activated charcoal does not appear to bring any benefit, and should therefore not be undertaken [36].

Treatment of the Muscarinic Syndrome

The mainstay of treatment of the muscarinic syndrome, characterized by diarrhea, urination, miosis, bronchorrhea, bradycardia, emesis, lacrimation, and salivation (DUMBELS) is atropine. The target of atropine therapy is resolution of bronchorrhea, as demonstrated by clear chest auscultation, and of bradycardia, with a heart rate greater than 80 bpm. Initial dosage should be ca 1-3 mg IV (0.02 mg/kg in children), with doses doubled each 3-5 minutes until sufficient atropinisation is obtained. The dosage required in pesticide intoxications, especially with suicidal intent, can be higher than is necessary in warfare nerve agent intoxications, probably due to the much larger amounts ingested. The failure to develop signs of atropinization after 2 mg of atropine is thought to be very suggestive of cholinesterase inhibitor poisoning.

Maintenance therapy with atropine is then 10 to 20% of the total initial dose, each hour, in a continuous infusion [10, 37-38]. Atropine dosage is then adjusted to clinical response in an intensive care setting, with progressive weaning as tolerated. Atropine therapy does not influence the amount of available active AChE, and is therefore a symptomatic therapy. Hence it must be maintained as long as the enzyme has not regenerated sufficiently to ensure proper function, either spontaneously or with antidotal oxime therapy. Recurrence of symptoms after cessation of atropine therapy can occur, making close observation for 48 hours post atropine cessation necessary.

Treatment of the Nicotinic Syndrome and Oxime Therapy

The nicotinic syndrome, characterized by mydriasis, tachycardia, weakness or paralysis, hypertension, hyperglycemia and fasciculations (MTWTF; days of the week) is atropine insensitive. Its treatment requires AChE reactivation, and can be obtained either spontaneously, by dissociation of the OP-AChE complex, by *de novo* synthesis of AChE or by oxime therapy.

Understanding the chemical mechanism of OP-AChE inactivation and oxime-induced reactivation is essential to proper understanding the basis of oxime therapy, its efficacy and its limitations. The initial AChE inhibition by OP is due to the phosphorylation of the active AChE serine site; this occurs by nucleophilic substitution, i.e. replacement of one of the substituents bonded to the phosphorous atom by the enzyme active site through formation of a covalent bond between the OP phosphorous and the AChE serine 203 hydroxyl oxygen [39]. This new covalent bond can be broken if another substituent with a higher affinity for the phosphorous atom, such as an oxime, is available. This yield a dephosphorylated and thus reactivated AChE, and a phosphorylated oxime that is less toxic than the original OP and is subsequently degraded and eliminated. The reactivation by oxime scavenging of the OP toxicant requires that the oxime have a greater affinity for the OP than AChE for the reaction to proceed in the intended direction. It is also necessary that the oxime have a lower affinity for AChE than the OP, as the oximes also have AChE-inhibiting properties and are known to cause respiratory failure and convulsions that can lead to death in experimental animals [40]. Such a non-compatibility of toxicant and antidote is exemplified in obidoxime treatment of soman-inhibited AChE, where the addition of obidoxime increases the AChE inhibition [41]. There are also reports of cardiovascular effects imputed to pralidoxime administration, s.a. hypertension and even recurrent asystole [38, 42].

As the reactivation reaction is of equimolar steochiometry, the amount of oxime must be comparable to the amount of OP to be neutralized, in order to avoid persistence of potentially toxic free oxime. As complete immediate AChE regeneration is not necessary for survival, the dose of oxime should thus be calculated to yield only subtotal regeneration. The large doses of OP involved in pesticide self-poisoning may also explain large doses of oximes required for their treatment [38, 43-44].

The oxime reactivation of the OP-inhibited AChE requires that there be a relatively labile bond between the inhibitor and the enzyme. If the OP phosphorus atom has a second bond susceptible to hydrolysis (*i.e.* a second good leaving group), the OP-AChE complex may react with ambient H_2O (non-enzymatic hydrolysis) replacing a P-O-R bond with a more electron-attracting P-OH bond; this stabilizes the bond between the OP phosphorous and the ser203 hydroxyl oxygen, making the nucleophilic substitution reaction of oxime-mediated ACHE reactivation impossible [45]. As previously mentioned, this stabilization of the ACHE-OP complex, which occurs in minutes with tabun and soman, hours with sarin or diethyl-OP, and days with or Vx, is called ageing, and once it has occurred, AChE activity recovery requires *de novo* synthesis.

Post-exposure oxime treatment of OP intoxication by a "nerve gas" has been well studied, and various toxicant /antidote couples have been tested [41]. Animal and *in vitro* studies have shown extremely different behavior of toxicants and antidotes. Five different oximes (methoxime, obidoxime, pralidoxime and the experimental HI-6 and HLo-7) were tested relative to soman, sarin, tabun, VX and GF. The efficacy of oxime therapy varies from VX intoxication, which can be treated effectively with all the tested oximes, to tabun poisoning, which resists all studied antidotes. However, most OP intoxications do not involve military chemicals, and hence the available data relative to their treatment is much scarcer; most studies do not differentiate between the different OP toxicants or even classes of OPs, and concern the administration of only one single type of oxime antidote. The efficacy of these oxime therapies in humans is not clear. Whereas Pawar [43] reports more favorable outcome in moderately severely OP intoxicated patients treated with higher doses of pralidoxime vs lower doses (2g bolus followed by 1g/h for 48 h vs resp 1g and 0.25 g/h), Eddlestone [38] reports no difference in morbidity-mortality between placebo and pralidoxime (2g bolus & 0.5 g/hr < 7 dy), even within more homogenous toxicant groups, in one of the rare clinical trials of oxime therapy where the toxicant identity is considered, albeit only by attribution to 2 broad classes. A 2005 Cochrane review [44] concluded that there is probable benefit of high-dose oxime therapy when administered promptly (<12 h post exposure) in confirmed cases of civilian diethyl – OP intoxication.

Treatment of OP-Induced Seizures

From a therapeutic standpoint, it is important to remember that there is in vivo and in vitro evidence that OP-induced seizures are not a direct consequence of AChE inhibition, but appear to be due to interaction of OP with acetylcholine-independent neuromodulation pathways, such as GABA and NMDA [46, 47, 48]. The difference in involved pathways is also invoked to explain the variability in seizure activity observed with various AChE inhibiting OP. Therefore, treatments targeting AChE-mediated effects are likely to be inefficient against the associated seizure activity. These must be addressed by drugs targeting the involved pathways, as the convulsions themselves contribute to immediate lethality. This is exemplified by the absence of anticonvulsive effect of atropine alone in soman intoxication [49]. Hence seizure control relies on action on non-cholinergic mechanisms. In clinical practice, OP-induced seizure treatment and prevention relies on benzodiazepines, namely diazepam, which should be administered promptly upon suspicion of OP intoxication, even in the absence of apparent convulsive activity. Propofol, which exerts not only

GABA-agonist, but NMDA-antagonist effects, has also shown protective effects relative to morbidity-mortality in animal studies [50]. As mentioned above, the OP-induced paralysis may mask the underlying convulsive activity, making its' diagnosis dependant on clinical suspicion alone, unless emergent electroencephalography is available.

Other Treatments for OP Intoxication

Some authors have reported intravenous alkalinisation with sodium bicarbonate as an adjunct to the treatment of OP poisoning. A Cochrane review [51] concluded nevertheless that there is insufficient data to recommend its routine use.

As OPs inhibit numerous cholinesterases, the OP-intoxicated patient may present with biochemical disturbances that will affect drug metabolisation; in particular, the inhibition of BuChE will interfere with suxamethonium, esmolol, procaine, prednisolone acetate and heroin metabolism, imposing added caution when the use of such substances is required or suspected (52,53).

Intermediate Syndrome Management

The intermediate syndrome is considered to be unrelated to a recurrence of muscarinic symptoms (17). Whereas no specific treatment is available, and spontaneous complete recovery is the norm, aggressive supportive treatment, including intubation and mechanical ventilation may be required (19).

OPIDN Management

As OPIDN appears at ca 1-3weeks post acute exposure, there is usually no more OP present making antidotal therapy useless. Treatment is thus purely supportive and symptomatic, with analgesia, spasmolytics (s.a.diazepam) and physical therapy regimens. Resolution without sequelae or persistent disability may occur [22].

CONCLUSIONS

Acute OP intoxication can be associated with many symptoms and clinical signs, including potentially life-threatening seizures and status epilepticus. The associated flaccid paralysis may mask the convulsive activity, which is then only detectable through EEG. Instead of being linked to the direct cholinergic toxidrome, OP-related seizures are more probably linked to the interaction of OP with acetylcholine-independent neuro-modulation pathways, such as GABA and NMDA.The importance of preventing, or, that failing, recognizing and treating OP-related seizures lies in that CNS damage from OP poisoning is thought to be due to the excitotoxicity of the seizure activity itself, rather than a direct toxic effect. Muscular weakness and paralysis occurring 1-4 days after the resolution of acute cholinergic toxidrome, « the intermediate syndrome » is usually not diagnosed until significant respiratory insufficiency has occurred; it is nevertheless a major cause of OP-induced morbidity and mortality and requires aggressive supportive treatment. The condition usually resolves spontaneously in 1-2 weeks.

OP intoxication treatment relies on prompt diagnosis, and specific and immediate treatment of the life-threatening symptoms. Since patients suffering from OP poisoning can secondarily expose care providers *via* contaminated skin, clothing, hair, or body fluids. EMS and hospital caregivers should be prepared to protect themselves with appropriate protective equipments, isolate such patients, and decontaminate them.

After prompt decontamination, the initial priority of patient management is an immediate ABCDE resuscitation approach, including aggressive respiratory support, since respiratory failure is the usual ultimate cause of death. The subsequent priority is initiating atropine therapy to oppose the muscarinic symptoms and diazepam to prevent or control seizures, with oximes added to enhance AChE activity recovery. Large doses of atropine and oximes may be necessary for poisoning due to suicidal ingestions of OP pesticides.

Despite the thousands of tons of OP produced, stockpiled and used mainly as pesticides all over the world, and despite the dramatic number of intoxications and deaths produced each year by these compounds, it has also to be emphasized that the level of scientific knowledge on their mechanisms of human toxicity and the extent of evidence on the medical treatment of the OP intoxicated patient is dramatically low. A tremendous effort of the scientific and medical community to fill theses gaps is required, as well as a worldwide political intent to limit the production and access to these products.

REFERENCES

[1]   Marrs TC. Organophosphates: history, chemistry, pharmacology. In: Karalliedde L, Feldman S, Henry J & Marrs T, Eds. Organophosphates and health. London. Imperial College Press 2001; 1-36.

[2]   Gunnell D, Eddleston M. Suicide by intentional ingestion of pesticides: a continuous tragedy in developing countries. Int J Epidemiol 2003;32:902-9

[3]   Dong X, Simon M.A. The epidemiology of organophosphate poisoning in urban Zimbabwe from 1995 to 2000. Int J Occup Environ Health 2001;7:333-8

[4]   Srinivas Rao C.H, Venkateswarlu V, Surender T, Eddleston M, Buckley NA. Insecticide poisoning in south India – opportunities for prevention and improved medical management. Trop Med Int Health 2005 ;10 :581-8

[5]   Jaga K, Dharmani C. The interrelation between organophosphate toxicity and the epidemiology of depression and suicide. Reviews Environ Health 2007; 22 :57-73

[6]   Eddleston M, Buckley NA, Eyer P, Dawson AH. Management of acute organophosphorus pesticide poisoning. Lancet 2008; 371:597-607

[7]   Edwards P. Factors influencing organophosphate toxicity in humans. In: Karalliedde L, Feldman S, Henry J & Marrs T, Eds. Organophosphates and health. London. Imperial College Press. 2001; 61-82

[8]   Sanchez-Guerra MA, Elizondo-Azuela G, Perez-herrera N, Borja-Alburto V, Quitanilla-Vega B. Participation of CYP1A2*1F polypmorphism in the susceptibility of neurological effects by organophosphate pesticide exposure. Epidemiology 2007; 18: S146

[9]   National Library of Medicine. Specialized Information Service: Chemical Warfare agents, ChemIDplus Advanced. http://chem.sis.nlm.nih.gov/chemidplus/chemidlite.jsp (accessed January 28, 2010).

[10]   Roberts DM, Aaron CK. Managing acute organophosphorus pesticide poisoning. BMJ 2007; 334: 629-634

[11]   Jokanovic M. Medical treatment of acute poisoning with organophosphorus and carbamate pesticides. Toxicol Lett 2009; 190: 107-115

[12]   Yurumez Y, Durukan P, Yavuz Y, Ikizceli I, Avsarogullari L, Ozkan S, Akdur O, Ozdemir C. Acute organophosphate poisoning in University Hospital emergency room patients. Internal Med 2007; 46: 965-969

[13]   Kamanyire R, Karalliedde L. Organophosphate toxicity and occupational exposure. Occup Med 2004; 54: 69-75

[14]   Okumura T, Takasu N, Ishimatsu S, Miyanoki S, Mitsuhashi A, Kumada K, Tanaka K, Hinohara S. Report of the 640 victims of the Tokyo subway sarin attack. Ann Emerg Med 1996; 28: 129-135

[15]   Tokuda Y, Kikuchi M, Takahashi O, Stein GH. Prehospital management of sarin nerve gas terrorism in urban settings: 10 years of progress after the Tokyo subway sarin attack. Resuscitation 2006; 68: 193-202

[16]   Gharahbaghian L, Bey T. Sarin and other nerve agents of the organophosphate class: properties, medical effects and management. Intern J Disaster Med 2003; 2: 103-108

[17]   Senanayake N, Karalliedde L. Neurotoxic effects of organophosphorus insecticides: an intermediate syndrome. NEJM 1987; 13: 761-763

[18]   Jayawardane P, Dawson A, Weerasinghe V, Karalliedde L, Buckley NA, Senanayake N. The spectrum of intermediate syndrome following acute organophosphate poisoning: a prospective cohort study from Sri Lanka. PLoS Med 2008; 5: 1143-1153

[19]   Yang CC, Deng JF. Intermediate syndrome following organophosphate insecticide poisoning. J Chin Med Assoc 2007; 70: 467-472

[20]   Moretto A, Lotti M. Poisoning by organophosphorus insecticides and sensory neuropathy. J Neurol Neurosurg Psychiatry 1998; 64:463-468

[21]   Emerick GL, Peccinini RG, de Oliveira GH. Organophosphorus-induced delayed neuropathy: A simple and efficient therapeutic strategy. Toxicol Lett 2009; [Epub ahead of print].

[22]   Abou-Donia MB, Lapadula DM. Mechanisms of organophosphorus ester-induced delayed neurotoxicity: type I and type II. Ann Rev Pharmacol Toxi 1990; 30: 405-440

[23]   Lader M. The effects of organophosphates on neuropsychiatric and psychological functioning. In: Karalliedde L, Feldman S, Henry J & Marrs T, Eds. Organophosphates and health. London. Imperial College Press. 2001; 175-198

[24]   Myhrer T. Neuronal structures involved in the induction and propagation of seizures caused by nerve agents: implications for medical treatment. Toxicology 2007; 239:1-14

[25]   Carpentier P, Foquin A, Dorandeu F, Lallement G. Delta activity as an early indicator for soman-induced brain damage : a review. NeuroToxicol 2001 ; 22 :299-315

[26]   Kim YB, Hur GH, Lee YS, Han BG, Shin S. A role of nitric oxide in organophosphate-induced convulsions. Environ Toxicol Pharmacol 1997; 3: 53-56

[27] Myhrer T, Andersen JM, Nguyen N, Aas P. Soman-induced convulsions in rats terminated with pharmacological agents after 45 min: neuropathology and cognitive performance. NeuroToxicol 2005; 26: 38-48

[28] Tuovinen K. Organophosphate-induced convulsions and prevention of neuropathological damages. Toxicology 2004; 196: 31-39

[29] Myhrer T, Skymoen LR, Aas P. Pharmacological agents, hippocampal EEG, and anticonvulsivant effects on soman-induced seizures in rats. Neurotoxico 2003; 24: 357-367

[30] Harrison P, Sheridan RD, Green AC, Scott IR, Tattersall JE. A guinea pig hippocampal slice model of organophosphate-induced seizure activity. J Pharmaco Exp Ther 2004; 310:678-686

[31] Aroniadou-Anderjaska V, Figueiredo T, Apland JP, Qashu F, Braga M. Primary brain targets of nerve agents: the role of the amygdalia in comparison to the hippocampus. Neurotoxicology. 2009;30:772-776.

[32] Apland JP, Aroniadou-Anderjaska V, Braga M. Soman induces ictogenesis in the amygdale and interictal activity in the hippocampus that are blocked by a GluR5 kainate receptor antagonist *in vitro*. Neuroscience 2009; 159: 380-389

[33] Jokanović M. Medical treatment of acute poisoning with organophosphorus and carbamate pesticides. Toxicol Lett 2009; 190: 107-15

[34] Davies JO, Eddleston M, Buckley NA. Predicting outcome in acute organophosphorus poisoning with a poison severity score or the Glasgow coma scale. Q J Med 2008; 101: 507-508

[35] Costa LG. Biomarker research in neurotoxicology: The role of mechanistic studies to bridge the gap between the laboratory and epidemiological investigations. Environ. Health. Perspect. 1996 ; 104 : 55-67

[36] Eddleston L *et al.* Multiple-dose activated charcoal in acute self-poisoning: a randomised controlled trial. The Lancet 2008 ; 371 : 579 – 587

[37] Baud F, Kayouka M, Houzé P. Mise au point sur le traitement des intoxications par les insecticides organophosphorés. Paris, France. Société Française de Médecine d'Urgence, 2009

[38] Eddleston M et al, Pralidoxime in acute organophosphorous insecticide poisonning- arandomised conrolled trial. PLoS Medicine 2009;6;e10000104

[39] Kwasnieski O, Verdier L, Malacria M, Derat E, Fixation of the two Tabun isomers in Acetylcholinesterase: a QM/MM study. J Phys Chem B 2009; 113: 10001-7

[40] Bartosova, L, Kamil K, Kuneseva G, Jun D, The acute toxicity of acetylcholinesterase reactivators in mice in relation to their structure. Neurotox Res 2006; 9: 291-296

[41] Kassa J, Review of oximes in the antidotal treatment of poisoning by organophosphorous nerve agents. J Toxicol 2002; 40: 803-816

[42] Scott RJ, Repeated asystole following PAM in organophosphate self-poisonning. Anaesth Intensive Care 1986 ; 14: 458-460

[43] Pawar, KS *et al.* Continuous pralidoxime infusion versus repeated bolus injection to treat organophosphorous pesticide poisoning: a randomized controlled trial. Lancet 2006; 368: 2136-41

[44] Buckley N, Eddleston M, Szinicz L. Oximes for acute organophosphate pesticide poisoning. Cochrane Database of Systematic Reviews 2005, Issue 1. CD005085. DOI: 10.1002/14651858. CD005085

[45] Auf Der Heide E. TSDR CSEM: Cholinesterase Inhibitors Including Insecticides and Chemical Warfare Nerve Agents, http://www.atsdr.cdc.gov/csem/cholinesterase; 2007

[46] Chebabo SR, Santos MD, Albuquerque EX. The organophosphate Sarin, at low concentrations, inhibits the evoked release of GABA in rat hippocampla slices. NeuroToxicology 1999; 20: 871-882

[47] Weissman BA, Raveh L. Therapy against organophosphate poisoning: the importance of antocholinergic drugs with antiglutamatergic properties. Toxicology and Applied Pharmacology 2008; 232: 351-358

[48] Raveh L *et al.* The involvement of the NMDA receptor complex in the protective effect of anticholinergic drugs against soman poisoning. NeuroToxicology 1999; 20: 551-560.

[49] Shih TM. Cholinergic actions of diazepam and atropine sulfate in soman poisoning. Brain Research Bulletin 1991; 26: 556-573

[50] Peterson SL, Purvis RS, Griffith JW. Anticonvulsant and neuroprotective effects of propofol in cholinergic status epilepticus, in "Treatment strategies for the NMDA component of organophosphorouos convulsions", appendix 3, DAMD17-01-1-0794 2005

[51] Roberts DM, Buckley N. Alkalinisation for organophosphorous pesticide poisoning. Cochrane database of systematic reviews 2005, issue 1 Art No.: CD004897. DOI: 10.1002/14641858.CD004897.pub2

[52] Karalliedde L, Henry J. The acute cholinergic syndrome. In: Karalliedde L, Feldman S, Henry J & Marrs T, Eds. Organophosphates and health. London. Imperial College Press 2001; pp 257 – 293

[53] Williams FM, Clinical significance of esterases. Clinical Pharmacokinetics 1985;10: 392-403.

CHAPTER 4

Organophosphate Toxicity Relating to Exposure Route and Type of Agent

Marloes J.A. Joosen[1,*], Marcel J. van der Schans[1], August B. Smit[2] and Herman P.M. van Helden[1]

[1]TNO Defence, Security and Safety, Department of Chemical Toxicology, Lange Kleiweg 137, 2288GJ, Rijswijk, The Netherlands and [2]Center for Neurogenomics and Cognitive Research, Free University, De Boelelaan 1085, 1081HV, Amsterdam, The Netherlands

Abstract: The current medical countermeasures for organophosphate (OP) poisoning are effective to a reasonable extent, yet, there is room for improvement. In this review, suspected causes of acute and long term-effects of OP-exposure and possible interventions will be discussed, in relation to the type of nerve agent and different exposure routes. Inhibition of AChE by organophosphates leads to excessive buildup of released acetylcholine (ACh) at cholinergic synapses resulting in a failure of neuromuscular transmission and leads to seizures followed by status epilepticus. Eventually, poisoning with OPs is likely to result in death or long-term neuronal deficits.

Although, the OP nerve agents soman and VX act *via* a similar mechanism, that is inhibition of AChE, the toxicological impact following exposure shows to be quite different. Whereas, toxic signs upon sc exposure to soman in general develop very rapidly with the presence of seizures, pc exposure to VX animals shows delayed development of clinical signs compared to sc soman exposure. Such differences in agent behavior put special demands on treatment.

Another important conclusion of the present study is that an effective life-saving treatment at short term, may not be sufficient to prevent long term cognition deficits. This implies that a more thorough understanding of the cause of such deficits is needed to design improved treatment strategies. Suppression of the inflammatory processes in seizure initiation and continuation and restoring impaired neurogenesis, the latter proposed as a cause of cognition deficits following soman exposure, could be starting points for improved treatment.

INTRODUCTION

Organophosphates

Organophosphates (OPs) are a group of chemicals that have many domestic and industrial uses. OPs still represent the largest class of insecticides and are responsible for a large number of poisonings, in particular in developing countries. Development of OP compounds into insecticides occurred in the late 1930s by the German scientist Dr. Gerhard Schrader. This research led to the discovery and development of nerve agents as chemical warfare agents (CWAs), such as Tabun, Sarin, Soman, and VX (see Fig. **1**). Due to their severe toxicity on humans most nations have signed the Geneva Protocol pledging never to use CWAs in military conflicts. However, this could not prevent that sarin was used by terrorists in attacks against the civilian populations in Japan in 1994, 1995. The target of such attacks by terrorist groups may include not only the civilian population, but also the armed forces.

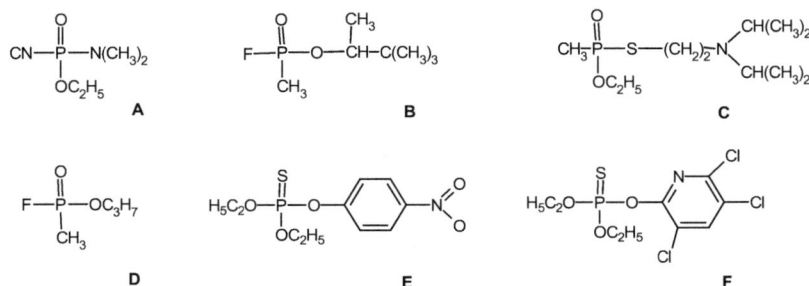

Figure 1: Chemical formulas of the most well-known nerve agents (A through D) and pesticides (E and F), organic esters of phosphoric acid. They possess a central phosphorous atom bound to two alkyl groups, a leaving group and oxygen or sulphur atom. A. Tabun (O-ethyl-N,N-dimethyl-phosphoramidocyanidate); B Soman (Pinacolylmethylphosphono-fluoridate); C. VX (O-ethyl-S-2-diisoprpylaminoethyl-methylphosphonothiolate) D. Sarin (Isopopylmethylphosphonofluoridate); E. Parathion; F. Chlorpyrifos

*****Address correspondence to Marloes Joosen**: TNO Defence, Security and Safety, Department of Chemical Toxicology, Lange Kleiweg 137, 2288GJ, Rijswijk, The Netherlands; Tel. +31 15 2843336; E-mail: marloes.joosen@tno.nl

Feng Ru Tang and Weng Keong Loke (Eds)

Researchers created many chemically modified OP compounds hoping to be able to find ones that would specifically target certain insect species, thereby limiting their unwanted effects in humans. However, when for example the OP insecticide parathion (Fig.. **1E**) was first employed as a replacement for the more toxic non-organophosphate DDT, a number of workers accustomed to handling parathion were killed. Another example, chlorpyrifos (Fig. **1 F**) is a pesticide that causes tens of thousands of deaths per year worldwide and OP pesticide self-poisoning is a major clinical problem, killing an estimated 200,000 people every year [1-2].

Because acute OP poisoning may induce severe toxicity, it requires immediate countermeasures. The change in threat scenarios regarding exposure to nerve agent in the past years demands a different approach for countermeasures than before. The probability of nerve agents being used on the battlefield is low, and exposures will most likely be unexpected or accidental. Consequently, people exposed will not have received pretreatment. Despite extensive research on medical countermeasures, treatment efficacy is far from optimal. A comprehensive understanding of the effects of OPs on the human body is needed to allow development of improved medical countermeasures to benefit people either exposed occupationally, through self harm or *via* deliberate release. In this review, suspected causes of acute and long term-effects of OP-exposure and possible interventions will be discussed, in relation to the type of nerve agent and different exposure routes.

TOXICITY OF ORGANOPHOSPHATES

Exposure Risks

Exposure to OP pesticides can occur *via* the oral, dermal or inhalation route. Oral dosing is mostly the result of accidental ingestion or in case of suicide attempts. The general population may also be chronically exposed to low doses by consumption of OP pesticide residues in food or as contaminant in drinking water. People working in production, transport, mixing, loading and application of pesticides are at highest risk for exposure, mostly *via* the dermal route [3-4]. With regard to nerve agents, the more volatile agents, soman, tabun and sarin, constitute both a vapour and a liquid hazard upon dispersion. In this case, toxic signs progress very rapidly due to inhalational exposure. Agents with lower volatility, such as VX, represent primarily a liquid hazard, and therefore skin contamination forms the highest risk. Toxicokinetics following skin exposure have shown to be highly variable and VX levels rise for several hours after a period of initial delay. In addition, VX is very persistent, because it hardly degrades and is difficult to wash off [5-6]. Such differences in agent behavior put special demands on treatment.

Seizure Development and Neurotoxicity

The main toxicological action of OPs, such as soman and VX, is exerted through irreversible inhibition of acetylcholinesterase (AChE), the key enzyme involved in cholinergic neurotransmission. The inhibition of AChE leads to excessive buildup of released acetylcholine (ACh) at cholinergic synapses resulting in a failure of neuromuscular transmission and leads to seizures followed by status epilepticus. Eventually, poisoning with OPs is likely to result in death or long-term neuronal deficits.

The mechanisms underlying OP neurotoxicity are subject to debate. Some evidence exists for direct neurotoxic effects of OPs, both from *in vitro* and *in vivo* studies. Several OPs have shown to possess cytotoxic activity in cultured neuroblastoma cells [7,8], rat hippocampal cell cultures [9] and in rat cortical neurons [10]. Other direct effects of OPs are disruption of polymerisation of microtubules [11], an altered sensitivity to glutamate excitotoxicity, and a decline in expression of synaptic proteins, indicating that OPs are able to directly induce synaptopathogenesis [12]. *In vivo*, low doses of OP, not causing acute toxicity, have shown to lead to subtle behavioral dysfunctions in rats [13-15]. In addition, inflammatory processes are implicated in initiation and continuation of seizures and following neurodegeneration [16-17]. These findings imply that OPs are capable of inducing neurotoxicity, largely independent from AChE inhibition, and this capacity seems to be different amongst OPs.

However, the toxicity following OP exposure is thought to be mainly mediated by ongoing seizure activity. Seizures appear to be generated *via* specific anatomical routes (Fig. 2). The piriform cortex is the first site to be activated in seizure propagation, and therefore identified as a key site for seizure initiation, followed by the amygdala, hippocampus, thalamus, cortical areas and striatum [18]. Accordingly, upon OP exposure, the most severe signs of neuropathology are located in these regions, indicating their involvement in seizure propagation [19].

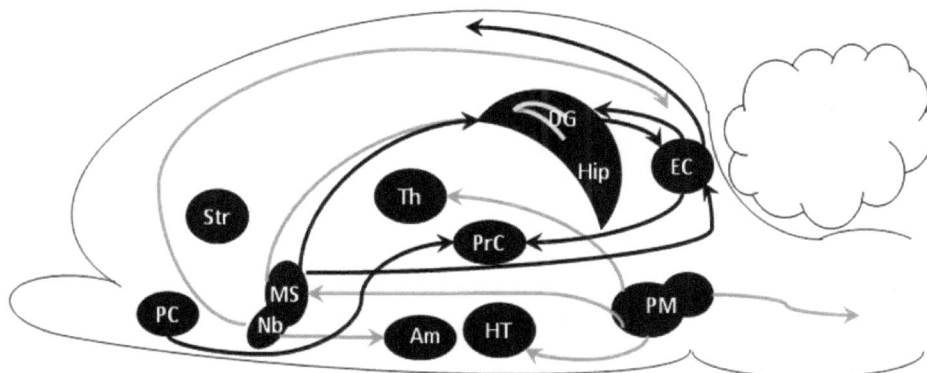

Figure 2: Schematic presentation of the main cholinergic (gray arrows) and seizure propagating (black arrows) pathways in a lateral view of the rodent brain. Neurons in the medial septum (MS) project to the hippocampus; neurons in the Nucleus Basalis (Nb) project to the Amygdala (Am) and to the Cortical region and neurons in the pontomesenphalon (PM) project to the hindbrain, Thalamus (Th), Hypothalamus (Ht) and basal forebrain (MS and Nb). Upon OP poisoning, the piriform cortex (PC) innervates the Perirhinal Cortex (PrC). The MS activates the hippocampus (Hip) and the Entorhinal Cortex (EC). The EC projects to the hippocampus *via* the perforant pathway, and to all cortical areas including motor areas. Adapted from Myhrer (2007) and Woolf (1991).

Two brain areas are identified as seizure controlling areas, *i.e.*, the substantia nigra and the area tempestas, which is located in the piriform cortex. Seizure modulation *via* the substantia nigra is only susceptible to treatment with GABAergic drugs, whereas in the area tempestas cholinergic, glutamatergic and GABAergic drugs are effective [20-22]. In the medial septal area, soman-induced seizures can be controlled by atropine [23-24]. Selective lesions of the area tempestas or medial septum are also effective in preventing soman-induced seizures [25]. The area tempestas and the medial septum have been proposed to cause hyperactivity in the hippocampal region in two ways: first, *via* direct cholinergic input, and second, *via* cholinergic input into the entorhinal cortex, which in turn activates the glutamatergic perforant path. *Via* the hippocampus, the entorhinal cortex innervates other cortical areas, including motor areas, thereby propagating epileptiform activity.

It is proposed that a 3-phased sequential recruitment of different neurotransmitter systems is involved in the initiation and maintenance of seizure activity [26]. The neurochemical event initiating seizure activity in susceptible neuronal circuits is the accumulation of ACh, characterized as the cholinergic phase [27-30]. During a transition phase, excitatory activity rapidly spreads and other neurotransmitter systems, such as the glutamatergic system, are recruited. At that moment, ACh levels return to normal, accompanied by increases in dopamine and GABA concentrations [26, 28, 31].

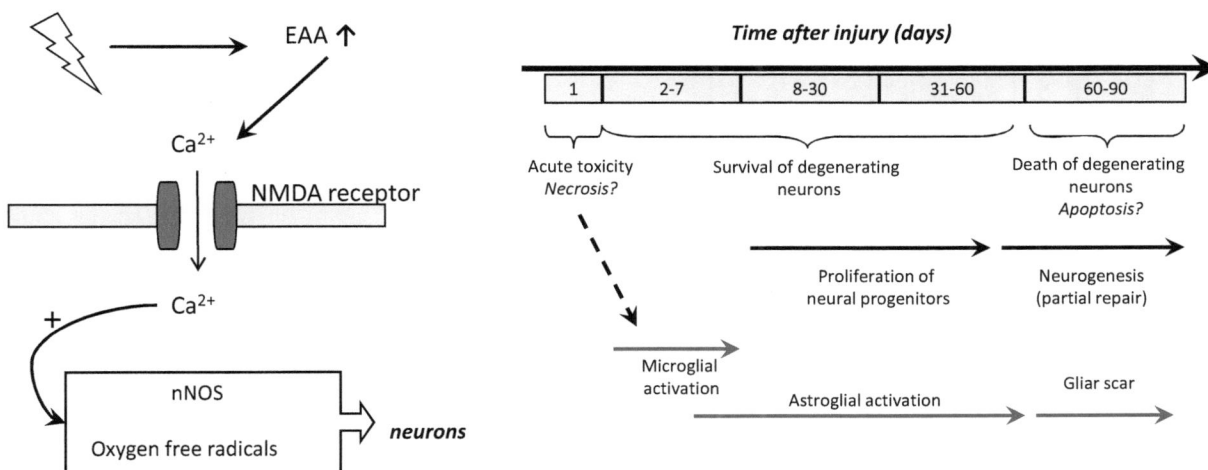

Figure 3: Excitotoxicity mediated by OP-induced seizures (left) and an overview of the CNS response to OP-induced neurotoxicity as proposed by Collombet *et al.* (2005) (right).

The excessive excitatory amino acid (EAA) release is thought to be the main mediator of OP-induced brain injury (Fig. **3**). Studies on epilepsy and OP-induces seizures revealed that 40 to 60 minutes of seizures are required to induce neuronal death [32-35]. The duration and intensity of seizures has shown to correlate well with the degree of neuropathology [19, 34-36]. The glutamate released as a result of ongoing seizures activates the postsynaptic NMDA receptors, leading to excessive calcium influx into neurons. This, in turn, triggers activation of proteolytic enzymes, phospholipases, neuronal NOS and it triggers free radical generation, resulting in neuronal damage. The assumed time course of events following OP-poisoning has been depicted by Collombet *et al.* (2005)[54] (Fig. **3**).

Effects on Neurogenesis and Cognition

OP poisoning initiates a period of acute toxicity, in which numerous cells die, after which microglial cells are activated peaking at day 3, followed by astroglial activation peaking at day 8 (Fig. **3**). These cells produce numerous cytokines, neutrophic- and growth factors which might contribute to the prolonged survival of degenerating neurons 3 to 60 days after soman exposure [37-38]. After returning to normal glial activity at days 30-60, a period of delayed toxicity is present, in which the damaged neurons slowly die, paralleled by glial scar formation and partial repair by neurogenesis. Although apoptotic cells are mostly absent, probably due to the rapidity and energy dependence of the process [39], degenerating cells resulting from soman-induced seizures show increased expression of proteins related to programmed cell death, indicating the presence of a hybrid form of cell death between apoptosis and necrosis [34].

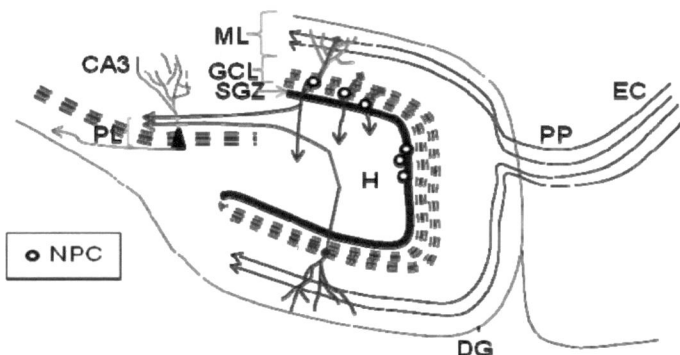

Figure 4: Illustration of neurogenesis in the adult dentate gyrus of the hippocampus. Neuronal progenitor cells (NPCs) are located in the subgranular zone (SGZ), which separates the granular layer (GCL) from the hilus (H). After differentiation of the NPCs into neurons in the SGZ, the neurons migrate into the GCL. Their dendrites project through the molecular layer (ML) and the axons project towards CA3 and the hilus. The dendrites receive input from the entorhinal cortex (EC) *via* the perforant path (PP). Adapted from Schinder and Gage (2004).

The long-term deficits as a consequence of OP exposure urge for understanding the mechanisms that might stimulate brain repair and mental health. In the past decade, it has become apparent that in specific parts of the adult brain new neurons are formed, a process termed neurogenesis [40-43]. Two main regions in the hippocampus, the subgranular zone (SGZ) and the dentate gyrus (DG) show prominent levels of neurogenesis (Fig. **4**). In these regions, newborn neurons undergo migration before they eventually mature [43]. Neural progenitor cells are distributed along the SGZ. In this region, they proliferate and differentiate, followed by a superficial migration into the GCL. The cell bodies remain in the granular cell layer, with their dendrites projecting through the molecular layer, and the axons projecting to the hilus and CA3 region [43-45].

The rate of neurogenesis is affected by several factors. Stress and aging suppress the levels of neurogenesis in the hippocampus [46-48]. Corticosterone injections also reduce the levels of hippocampal cell proliferation [49]. Physical activity is associated with increases in neurogenesis [50]. A role for neurogenesis has been implicated in hippocampal learning and memory [51-52]. It has been shown that neurogenesis in the SGZ of rodents is induced by brain injury resulting from seizures or ischemia shortly after injury, also in OP poisoning [53-57].

Different neurotransmitters, among which glutamate, acetycholine and serotonin, have been implicated in the regulation of neurogenesis. They might form entry points for pharmacological invervention. NMDA receptor activation reduces neurogenesis, whereas lesion of the perforant path, reducing the glutamatergic input from the

Entorhinal cortex into the hippocampus, showed to enhance neurogenesis [58-59]. Selective serotonin reuptake inhibitors, used as anti-depressants (*e.g.* fluoxetine), and atypical anti-psychotics (*e.g.* olanzapine) have shown to increase neurogenesis [60-63]. Damage to the cholinergic circuitry projecting to the hippocampus has been shown to suppress neurogenesis [64-66], whereas the reversible AChE inhibitor donepezil enhanced neurogenesis [67]. So, both brain injury resulting from seizures, as well as cholinergic impairment following OP poisoning might interfere with neurogenesis and accordingly with cognition. If so, restoration or pharmacological stimulation of neurogenesis might be an attractive approach for the treatment of long-term degenerative processes culminating in cognition deficits. We recently investigated this opportunity for treatment improvement in OP poisoning [69].

For that purpose, we employed a seizure model in the rat using the nerve agent soman (200 ug/kg sc). An effective and life saving treatment with the oxime HI-6 (125 mg/kg i.p. 30 minutes before soman) and atropine (1 mg/kg im 1 minute after soman) led to a high survival rate of 70%. Seizures were only present for less than 10 minutes on average, which was accompanied by a huge increase in extracellular acetylcholine levels for 40 minutes in the striatum of these animals (Fig. 5). At 24 hours after poisoning, no histological brain injury was observed. At 8 weeks after exposure, the soman-poisoned animals had a significantly impaired learning curve in the morris water maze, in spite of the absence of visually detectable brain injury. Their memory retrieval showed to be unaffected. As seizures were only present for a short time the cognitive deficits may not have resulted from excitotoxicity, but probably due to an imbalance in cholinergic input into the dentate gyrus, implicating that soman exposure undermines the neurogenesis process. In the same study, it was aimed to enhance neurogenesis by means of subchronic treatment with the antipsychotic olanzapine, that has shown to increase neurogenesis [60]. It appeared that neurogenesis was not enhanced by this drug at 8 weeks after soman exposure and was not effective in restoring cognitive deficits in this study. This leaves open that other doses or drugs might increase neurogenesis in such a way that it could improve cognition. To this end, it is recommended to test growth factors [68] and anticholinesterases such as physostigmine or galantamine when cognition deficits show up [67]. In addition, physical exercise might help to restore the balance in neurogenesis in the DG of the, physical exercise might help to restore the balance in neurogenesis in the DG of the hippocampus [50].

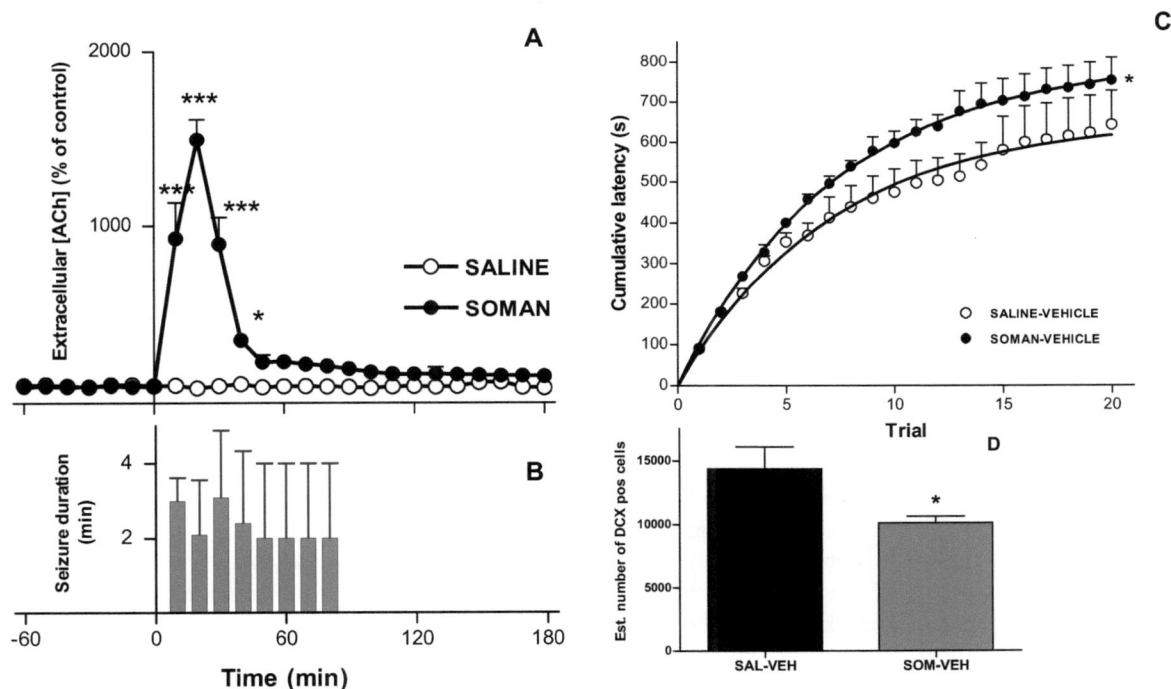

Figure 5: A. Extracellular ACh levels in the striatum of rats after saline (n=4, open dots)- or soman exposure (n=5, closed dots). (soman: 200 µg/kg s.c., t=0, pretreatment with 125 mg/kg HI-6 i.p. at t= -30 min; treatment with 16 mg/kg AS i.m. at t=1 min) are shown. Significant (*, p<0.05, two-way-ANOVA followed by Bonferoni's post-hoc test) elevation of ACh levels is present at 10-40 minutes after soman exposure. B Seizure duration in minutes (mean +/- SEM) of the soman-poisoned animals

synchronized with the 10-min periods of the ACh sampling. C Performance in Morris water maze 8 weeks after soman exposure. Average cumulative seconds to reach the platform (mean +/- SEM). Soman-intoxicated animals used significantly more time to find the platform than saline-injected animals (Y_{max},). D. Estimated numbers of DCX-positive cells in different treatment groups determined by stereological quantification. The number of DCX- positive cells after soman poisoning is significantly lower than that of control animals. Figures adapted and with permission from Joosen *et al.* 2009.

Toxicological Profiles

Although both soman and VX act *via* a similar mechanism, that is inhibition of AChE, the toxicological impact following exposure shows to be quite different. Whereas toxic signs upon sc exposure to soman in general develop very rapidly with the presence of seizures (Fig. **6A**), after pc exposure to VX, animals show a delay in development of clinical signs compared to sc soman exposure. In addition, only one third of animals show seizures on their EEG [5,69]. The other animals show a decline in EEG power, which was associated to ischemia (Fig. **6B**). A possible explanation may be the difference in distribution of both agents due to their chemical structures on the one hand, and the exposure route on the other hand. Since the type and number of binding sites for soman and VX are assumed to be the same, the gradual entrance into the circulation of VX from the skin depot and its high persistence in the circulation may increase the chance for VX to encounter binding sites before entering the brain. This indicates that VX is more confined to the peripheral compartment, and that soman predominantly acts in the CNS. Such differential toxicological profiles have implications for timing and type of treatment. A schematic overview of these differential toxicological profiles and possible interventions is proposed in Fig. **7**.

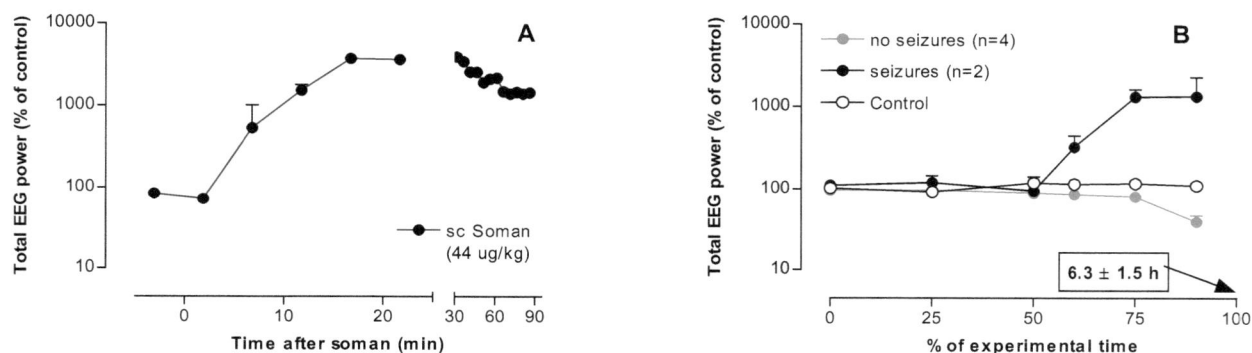

Figure 6: Seizure development represented by EEG Total Power increase after sc soman exposure (n=6) (A) and pc VX exposure (B). The EEG power is plotted on a real-time scale, and because of large interindividual differences the EEG after pc exposure to VX is plotted on a relative time scale, 100% averages 6.3 ± 1.5 hours.

Pharmacological intervention in case of OP exposure is maximally effective during different phases of poisoning. Prophylaxis with pyridostigmine and physostigmine is only effective before, and during the initial phase of poisoning, when AChE is not yet fully inhibited. Restoration of AChE activity by oximes is most efficacious in the initial phase of poisoning, in particular in case of rapid of soman-inhibited AChE. Antimuscarinic treatment by atropine counteracts the effect of accumulating ACh and is therefore also indicated during the acute phase of poisoning. However, atropine is not fully effective in preventing seizure development, therefore the culmination of seizures by anticonvulsants such as diazepam and midazolam is also indicated during the acute phase. The resulting neurotoxicity in this phase of toxicity is probably counteracted by NMDA antagonists, such as MK 801, or by drugs showing both antimuscarinic and anti-. glutamatergic activity, such as procyclidine Nevertheless, available data have shown that such treatments cannot fully prevent brain injury or cognitive deficits.

We have not yet investigated long-term effects after pc exposure to VX. It might be anticipated that a decrease in respiratory minute volume (RMV) and heart rate result in ischemia [69]. Ischemia induces brain injury, which is associated with cognitive decline [70]. The prevention of ischemic injury is probably best accomplished by atropine and oximes, which can protect the PNS from excessive levels of ACh. The results imply that apart from diminishing seizure activity, stabilization of the cholinergic pathway that regulates neurogenesis in the hippocampus, and prevention of ischemic injury might be additional targets to prevent long-term cognition deficits (Fig. 7).

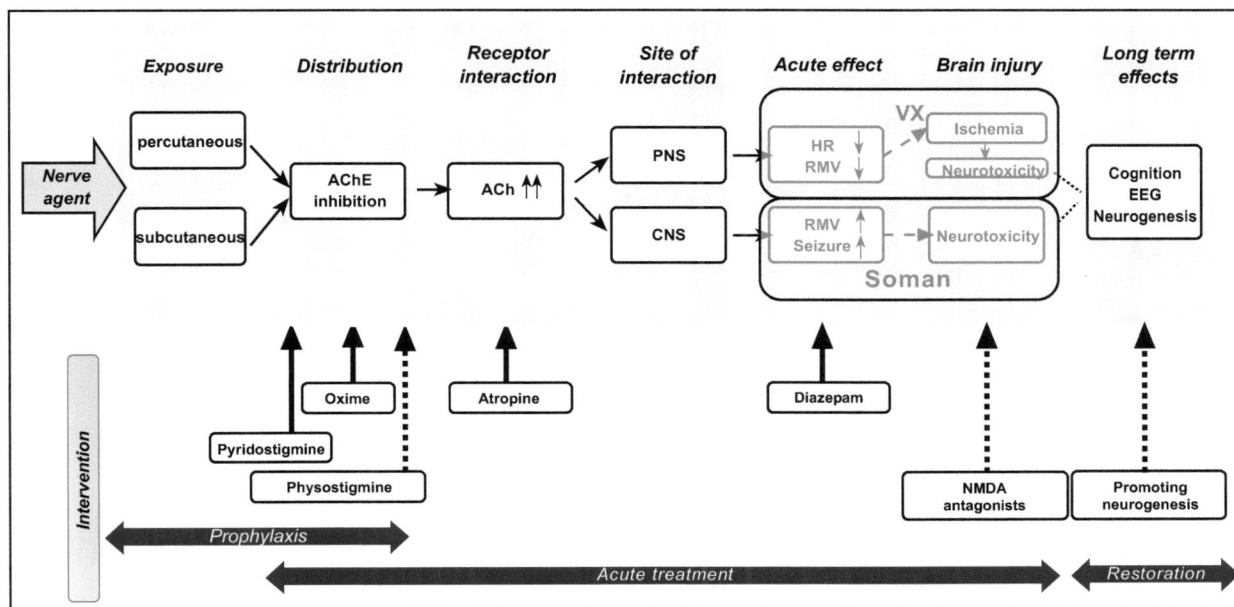

Figure 7: Overview of differential nerve agent effects and possible interventions. The subcutaneous route for soman represents an approximation of the inhalation route regarding toxicokinetics and effects. Vertical grey arrows indicate current countermeasures in use, dotted grey ones indicate novel countermeasures. See text for further explanation.

CONCLUSION

The toxicological profiles of sc soman exposure and pc VX exposure showed to be very different and accordingly demand a very different treatment approach. In particular, timing of treatment is implicated as an important issue in both cases. Soman exposure requires rapid treatment, directly aimed at restoring AChE activity and terminating seizure activity, whereas pc VX exposure requires repeated treatment on appearance of clinical signs to preserve vital functions, until all agents have entered the circulation and has been hydrolyzed.

The results from the VX experiments are useful to the clinical practice of OP insecticide poisoning, because of their similar persistence in the body. Another important conclusion of the present study is that an effective life-saving treatment at short term, may not be sufficient to prevent long term cognition deficits. This implies that a more thorough understanding of the cause of such deficits is needed to design improved treatment strategies. Suppression of the inflammatory processes in seizure initiation and continuation and restoring impaired neurogenesis, the latter proposed as a cause of cognition deficits following soman exposure, could be starting points for improved treatment.

REFERENCES

[1]   Eddleston M, Eyer P, Worek F, Mohamed F, Senarathna L, Von Meyer L, Juszczak E, Hittarage A, Azhar S, Dissanayake W, Sheriff MH, Szinicz L, Dawson AH, Buckley NA. Differences between organophosphorus insecticides in human self-poisoning: a prospective cohort study. Lancet 2005; 366: 1452-1459.
[2]   Eyer P. The role of oximes in the management of organophosphorus pesticide poisoning. Toxicol Rev 2003; 22: 165-190.
[3]   Costa LG, Giordano G, Guizzetti M, Vitalone A. Neurotoxicity of pesticides: a brief review. Front Biosci 2008; 13: 1240-1249.
[4]   Costa LG. Current issues in organophosphate toxicology. Clin Chim Acta 2006; 366: 1-13.
[5]   van der Schans MJ, Lander BJ, van der WH, Langenberg JP, Benschop HP. Toxicokinetics of the nerve agent (+/-)-VX in anesthetized and atropinized hairless guinea pigs and marmosets after intravenous and percutaneous administration. Toxicol Appl Pharmacol 2003; 191: 48-62.

[6]   Sidell FR. Nerve agents.1997; 129-180.

[7]   Carlson K,Ehrich M. Distribution of SH-SY5Y human neuroblastoma cells in the cell cycle following exposure to organophosphorus compounds. J Biochem Mol Toxicol 2008; 22: 187-201.

[8]   Carlson K, Jortner BS, Ehrich M. Organophosphorus compound-induced apoptosis in SH-SY5Y human neuroblastoma cells. Toxicol Appl Pharmacol 2000; 168: 102-113.

[9]   Bahrami F, Yousefpour M, Mehrani H, Golmanesh L, Sadraee SH, Khoshbaten A, Asgari A. Type of cell death and the role of acetylcholinesterase activity in neurotoxicity induced by paraoxon in cultured rat hippocampal neurons. Acta Biol Hung 2009; 60: 1-13.

[10]   Wang Y, Weiss MT, Yin J, Tenn CC, Nelson PD, Mikler JR. Protective effects of N-methyl-D-aspartate receptor antagonism on VX-induced neuronal cell death in cultured rat cortical neurons. Neurotox Res 2008; 13: 163-172.

[11]   Grigoryan H, Lockridge O. Nanoimages show disruption of tubulin polymerization by chlorpyrifos oxon: implications for neurotoxicity. Toxicol Appl Pharmacol 2009; 240: 143-148.

[12]   Munirathinam S, Bahr BA. Repeated contact with subtoxic soman leads to synaptic vulnerability in hippocampus. J Neurosci Res 2004; 77: 739-746.

[13]   Prendergast MA, Terry AV, Jr., Buccafusco JJ. Chronic, low-level exposure to diisopropylfluorophosphate causes protracted impairment of spatial navigation learning. Psychopharmacology (Berl) 1997; 129: 183-191.

[14]   Verma SK, Kumar V, Gill KD. An acetylcholinesterase-independent mechanism for neurobehavioral impairments after chronic low level exposure to dichlorvos in rats. Pharmacol Biochem Behav 2009; 92: 173-181.

[15]   Nieminen SA, Lecklin A, Heikkinen O, Ylitalo P. Acute behavioural effects of the organophosphates sarin and soman in rats. Pharmacol Toxicol 1990; 67: 36-40.

[16]   Dhote F, Peinnequin A, Carpentier P, Baille V, Delacour C, Foquin A, Lallement G, Dorandeu F. Prolonged inflammatory gene response following soman-induced seizures in mice. Toxicology 2007; 238: 166-176.

[17]   Fabene PF, Navarro MG, Martinello M, Rossi B, Merigo F, Ottoboni L, Bach S, Angiari S, Benati D, Chakir A, Zanetti L, Schio F, Osculati A, Marzola P, Nicolato E, Homeister JW, Xia L, Lowe JB, McEver RP, Osculati F, Sbarbati A, Butcher EC, Constantin G. A role for leukocyte-endothelial adhesion mechanisms in epilepsy. Nat Med 2008; 14: 1377-1383.

[18]   Zimmer LA, Ennis M, el Etri M, Shipley MT. Anatomical localization and time course of Fos expression following soman-induced seizures. J Comp Neurol 1997; 378: 468-481.

[19]   McDonough JH, Jr., Dochterman LW, Smith CD, Shih TM. Protection against nerve agent-induced neuropathology, but not cardiac pathology, is associated with the anticonvulsant action of drug treatment. Neurotoxicology 1995; 16: 123-132.

[20]   Gale K. Progression and generalization of seizure discharge: anatomical and neurochemical substrates. Epilepsia 1988; 29 Suppl 2: S15-S34.

[21]   Myhrer T, Nguyen NH, Enger S, Aas P. Anticonvulsant effects of GABA(A) modulators microinfused into area tempestas or substantia nigra in rats exposed to soman. Arch Toxicol 2006; 80: 502-507.

[22]   Myhrer T, Enger S, Aas P. Anticonvulsant efficacy of drugs with cholinergic and/or glutamatergic antagonism microinfused into area tempestas of rats exposed to soman. Neurochem Res 2008; 33: 348-354.

[23]   Denoyer M, Lallement G, Collet A, Pernot-Marino I, Sereno D, Blanchet G. Influence of medial septal cholinoceptive cells on c-Fos-like proteins induced by soman. Brain Res 1992; 592: 157-162.

[24]   Lallement G, Denoyer M, Collet A, Pernot-Marino I, Baubichon D, Monmaur P, Blanchet G. Changes in hippocampal acetylcholine and glutamate extracellular levels during soman-induced seizures: influence of septal cholinoceptive cells. Neurosci Lett 1992; 139: 104-107.

[25]   Myhrer T, Enger S, Aas P. Anticonvulsant effects of damage to structures involved in seizure induction in rats exposed to soman. Neurotoxicology 2007; 28: 819-828.

[26]   Shih TM, McDonough JH, Jr. Neurochemical mechanisms in soman-induced seizures. J Appl Toxicol 1997; 17: 255-264.

[27]   Lallement G, Carpentier P, Collet A, Baubichon D, Pernot-Marino I, Blanchet G. Extracellular acetylcholine changes in rat limbic structures during soman-induced seizures. Neurotoxicology 1992; 13: 557-567.

[28]   Fosbraey P, Wetherell JR, French MC. Neurotransmitter changes in guinea-pig brain regions following soman intoxication. J Neurochem 1990; 54: 72-79.

[29]   Tonduli LS, Testylier G, Marino IP, Lallement G. Triggering of soman-induced seizures in rats: multiparametric analysis with special correlation between enzymatic, neurochemical and electrophysiological data. J Neurosci Res 1999; 58: 464-473.

[30]   Bueters TJ, Groen B, Danhof M, IJzerman AP, van Helden HP. Therapeutic efficacy of the adenosine A1 receptor agonist N6-cyclopentyladenosine (CPA) against organophosphate intoxication. Arch Toxicol 2002; 76: 650-656.

[31]   Liu DD, Ueno E, Ho IK, Hoskins B. Evidence that alterations in gamma-aminobutyric acid and acetylcholine in rat striata and cerebella are not related to soman-induced convulsions. J Neurochem 1988; 51: 181-187.

[32]   Fujikawa DG. Prolonged seizures and cellular injury: understanding the connection. Epilepsy Behav 2005; 7 Suppl 3: S3-11.

[33]   Shih TM, Koviak TA, Capacio BR. Anticonvulsants for poisoning by the organophosphorus compound soman: pharmacological mechanisms. Neurosci Biobehav Rev 1991; 15: 349-362.

[34]   Baille V, Clarke PG, Brochier G, Dorandeu F, Verna JM, Four E, Lallement G, Carpentier P. Soman-induced convulsions: the neuropathology revisited. Toxicology 2005; 215: 1-24.

[35]   Carpentier P, Foquin A, Rondouin G, Lerner-Natoli M, de Groot DM, Lallement G. Effects of atropine sulphate on seizure activity and brain damage produced by soman in guinea-pigs: ECoG correlates of neuropathology. Neurotoxicology 2000; 21: 521-540.

[36]   Carpentier P, Foquin A, Dorandeu F, Lallement G. Delta activity as an early indicator for soman-induced brain damage: a review. Neurotoxicology 2001; 22: 299-315.

[37]   Lallement G, Baille V, Baubichon D, Carpentier P, Collombet JM, Filliat P, Foquin A, Four E, Masqueliez C, Testylier G, Tonduli L, Dorandeu F. Review of the value of huperzine as pretreatment of organophosphate poisoning. Neurotoxicology 2002; 23: 1-5.

[38]   Liberto CM, Albrecht PJ, Herx LM, Yong VW, Levison SW. Pro-regenerative properties of cytokine-activated astrocytes. J Neurochem 2004; 89: 1092-1100.

[39]   Nicotera P,Leist M. Energy supply and the shape of death in neurons and lymphoid cells. Cell Death Differ 1997; 4: 435-442.

[40]   Eriksson PS, Perfilieva E, Bjork-Eriksson T, Alborn AM, Nordborg C, Peterson DA, Gage FH. Neurogenesis in the adult human hippocampus. Nat Med 1998; 4: 1313-1317.

[41]   Gross CG. Neurogenesis in the adult brain: death of a dogma. Nat Rev Neurosci 2000; 1: 67-73.

[42]   Kuhn HG, Dickinson-Anson H, Gage FH. Neurogenesis in the dentate gyrus of the adult rat: age-related decrease of neuronal progenitor proliferation. J Neurosci 1996; 16: 2027-2033.

[43]   Schinder AF, Gage FH. A hypothesis about the role of adult neurogenesis in hippocampal function. Physiology (Bethesda) 2004; 19: 253-261.

[44]   Hastings NB, Gould E. Rapid extension of axons into the CA3 region by adult-generated granule cells. J Comp Neurol 1999; 413: 146-154.

[45]   Hastings NB, Seth MI, Tanapat P, Rydel TA, Gould E. Granule neurons generated during development extend divergent axon collaterals to hippocampal area CA3. J Comp Neurol 2002; 452: 324-333.

[46]   Heine VM, Maslam S, Zareno J, Joels M, Lucassen PJ. Suppressed proliferation and apoptotic changes in the rat dentate gyrus after acute and chronic stress are reversible. Eur J Neurosci 2004; 19: 131-144.

[47]   Kempermann G, Kuhn HG, Gage FH. Experience-induced neurogenesis in the senescent dentate gyrus. J Neurosci 1998; 18: 3206-3212.

[48]   Westenbroek C, Den Boer JA, Veenhuis M, Ter Horst GJ. Chronic stress and social housing differentially affect neurogenesis in male and female rats. Brain Res Bull 2004; 64: 303-308.

[49]   Cameron HA,Gould E. Adult neurogenesis is regulated by adrenal steroids in the dentate gyrus. Neuroscience 1994; 61: 203-209.

[50]   Van Praag H, Kempermann G, Gage FH. Running increases cell proliferation and neurogenesis in the adult mouse dentate gyrus. Nat Neurosci 1999; 2: 266-270.

[51]   Dobrossy MD, Drapeau E, Aurousseau C, Le Moal M, Piazza PV, Abrous DN. Differential effects of learning on neurogenesis: learning increases or decreases the number of newly born cells depending on their birth date. Mol Psychiatry 2003; 8: 974-982.

[52]   Dupret D, Fabre A, Dobrossy MD, Panatier A, Rodriguez JJ, Lamarque S, Lemaire V, Oliet SH, Piazza PV, Abrous DN. Spatial learning depends on both the addition and removal of new hippocampal neurons. PLoS Biol 2007; 5: e214-

[53]   Emsley JG, Mitchell BD, Kempermann G, Macklis JD. Adult neurogenesis and repair of the adult CNS with neural progenitors, precursors, and stem cells. Prog Neurobiol 2005; 75: 321-341.

[54]   Collombet JM, Four E, Bernabe D, Masqueliez C, Burckhart MF, Baille V, Baubichon D, Lallement G. Soman poisoning increases neural progenitor proliferation and induces long-term glial activation in mouse brain. Toxicology 2005; 208: 319-334.

[55]   Parent JM. Adult neurogenesis in the intact and epileptic dentate gyrus. Prog Brain Res 2007; 163: 529-540.

[56]   Wiltrout C, Lang B, Yan Y, Dempsey RJ, Vemuganti R. Repairing brain after stroke: a review on post-ischemic neurogenesis. Neurochem Int 2007; 50: 1028-1041.

[57]   Sharp FR, Liu J, Bernabeu R. Neurogenesis following brain ischemia. Brain Res Dev Brain Res 2002; 134: 23-30.

[58]   Cameron HA, McEwen BS, Gould E. Regulation of adult neurogenesis by excitatory input and NMDA receptor activation in the dentate gyrus. J Neurosci 1995; 15: 4687-4692.

[59]   Nacher J, Alonso-Llosa G, Rosell DR, McEwen BS. NMDA receptor antagonist treatment increases the production of new neurons in the aged rat hippocampus. Neurobiol Aging 2003; 24: 273-284.

[60]   Kodama M, Fujioka T, Duman RS. Chronic olanzapine or fluoxetine administration increases cell proliferation in hippocampus and prefrontal cortex of adult rat. Biol Psychiatry 2004; 56: 570-580.

[61]   Wakade CG, Mahadik SP, Waller JL, Chiu FC. Atypical neuroleptics stimulate neurogenesis in adult rat brain. J Neurosci Res 2002; 69: 72-79.

[62]   Paizanis E, Hamon M, Lanfumey L. Hippocampal neurogenesis, depressive disorders, and antidepressant therapy. Neural Plast 2007; 2007: 1-7.

[63]   Wang HD, Dunnavant FD, Jarman T, Deutch AY. Effects of antipsychotic drugs on neurogenesis in the forebrain of the adult rat. Neuropsychopharmacology 2004; 29: 1230-1238.

[64]   Cooper-Kuhn CM, Winkler J, Kuhn HG. Decreased neurogenesis after cholinergic forebrain lesion in the adult rat. J Neurosci Res 2004; 77: 155-165.

[65]   Van der Borght K, Mulder J, Keijser JN, Eggen BJ, Luiten PG, Van der Zee EA. Input from the medial septum regulates adult hippocampal neurogenesis. Brain Res Bull 2005; 67: 117-125.

[66]   Kotani S, Yamauchi T, Teramoto T, Ogura H. Pharmacological evidence of cholinergic involvement in adult hippocampal neurogenesis in rats. Neuroscience 2006; 142: 505-514.

[67]   Kotani S, Yamauchi T, Teramoto T, Ogura H. Donepezil, an acetylcholinesterase inhibitor, enhances adult hippocampal neurogenesis. Chem Biol Interact 2008; 175: 227-230.

[68]   Collombet JM, Four E, Burckhart MF, Masqueliez C, Bernabe D, Baubichon D, Herodin F, Lallement G. Effect of cytokine treatment on the neurogenesis process in the brain of soman-poisoned mice. Toxicology 2005; 210: 9-23.

[69]   Joosen MJ, van der Schans MJ, van Helden HP. Percutaneous exposure to VX: clinical signs, effects on brain acetylcholine levels and EEG. Neurochem Res 2008; 33: 308-317.

[70]   Bendel O, Bueters T, von Euler M, Ove OS, Sandin J, von Euler G. Reappearance of hippocampal CA1 neurons after ischemia is associated with recovery of learning and memory. J Cereb Blood Flow Metab 2005; 25:1586-95.

CHAPTER 5

Therapeutic Effects of Drug Combinations Targeting Muscarinic and Adrenoreceptors during Soman Poisoning

Weng Keong Loke[*] and Lai Kwan Ho

Defence Medical and Environmental Research Institute, DSO National Laboratories, 11 Stockport Road, Singapore 117605

Abstract: Soman, a potent acetylcholinesterase inhibitor, induces accumulation of acetylcholine at the neural synapses resulting in overstimulation of the cholinergic system. At lethal concentrations, Soman-induced seizures progress rapidly into status epilepticus, which if not terminated, will lead to eventual death or profound brain damage amongst survivors. The current diazepam anticonvulsant could stop seizures when administrated early but its efficacy diminishes rapidly when applied late post seizures. Increasing diazepam dosage to compensate for reduction in anticonvulsant potency enhances nerve agent-induced respiratory depression. Research is on-going to identify alternate neuroprotection options for managing established and refractory status epilepticus without increasing respiratory difficulties amongst nerve agent casualties. In this chapter, a review of the various neuroprotection options that have been investigated as alternatives to diazepam in the last decade is presented. In addition, we have also provided a comprehensive report on neuroprotective actions achieved with a combined administration of clonidine and atropine sulfate in Soman poisoned animals with status epilepticus. Clonidine, an α_2-adrenergic agonist, acts on post-synaptic heteroreceptors to exert pre-synaptic inhibition on release of acetylcholine while atropine sulphate, as a muscarinic antagonist, blocks cholinergic activation of post-synaptic muscarinic receptors. By targeting the central cholinergic system with this synergistic drug combination, besides enhancing animal survival, rapid seizure arrest was achieved with early administration while functional neuroprotection was observed in animals undergoing established status epilepticus. Interestingly, neuroprotection was achieved despite the continued presence of seizures, when it was applied during established status epilepticus and its effect was much higher than that afforded by diazepam. Inclusion of clonidine was vital for preventing atropine induced lethal ventricular arrhythmias in hypoxic animals when treatment was given late. This finding may be useful for reviewing the current perceived roles of central cholinergic and glutamatergic systems in maintaining established status epilepticus, which has directed much of current research for new neuroprotection options towards the glutamate system.

NEUROTOXIC EFFECTS OF NERVE AGENTS

Nerve agents exert their effect through irreversible inhibition of the nerve enzyme, acetylcholinesterase (AChE) [1,2]. Inhibition of AChE will result in accumulation of acetylcholine (ACh) at neural synapses to produce depolarisation block, hypersecretions, fasciculations, tremor, motor convulsions and respiratory distress [3]. From both experimental animals and recorded instances of accidental human exposures to lethal doses of nerve agents, rapid induction of electrographic seizures was typically observed within 3-4 minutes of inhalational exposure. The type of seizures that occurs after a lethal dose of nerve agent is termed as generalised convulsive status epilepticus (GCSE), the most common and most potentially damaging form of status epilepticus(SE). It is clinically defined as 30 minutes of continuous tonic-clonic seizure, with full loss of consciousness that leads to a wide spectrum of clinical symptoms [4]. From animal studies, nerve agent-induced status epilepticus is self-sustaining in animals that survived the intoxicated but not given anticonvulsants promptly [5]. In our study, all rats pretreated (-30 minutes) with a protective dose of HI-6 oxime (125 mg/kg; i.p.) prior to a lethal dose of Soman (1.6 x LD_{50}; 176 μg/kg, subcutaneous) injection developed electrocorticographic (EEG) seizures after a latency of (5.9 ± 0.2) min [6]. Similar to previous studies with other animal models and clinical reports of status epilepticus, the seizures progressed over 5-phases with a brief Phase III entering rapidly into Phase IV after the first hour of seizure (Fig. **1**) [7]. Most seizures recordings remained in Phase IV for the first 4 hours of recording before the inter-ictal duration slowly lengthens to enter into Phase V of status epilepticus. The latter phase is usually observed amongst intoxicated animals at 24 hours post seizures onset.

*****Address correspondence to Dr Weng Keong Loke:** Defence Medical and Environmental Research Institute, DSO National Laboratories, 11 Stockport Road, Singapore 117605; Tel: 65-68712885; E-mail: *lwengkeo@dso.org.sg*

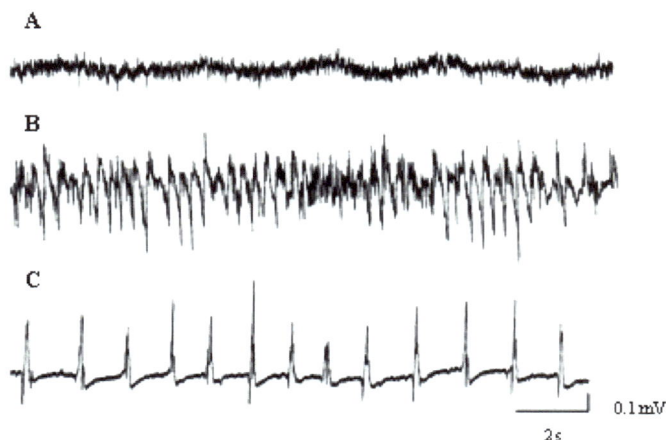

Figure 1: Representative of EEG patterns of a Soman poisoned rat; (A) baseline, (B) several minutes post seizure onset, (C) regular spikes of seizure activity after 4 hours to 24 hours.

In comparison, motor convulsions were often observed prior to appearance of EEG seizures and became most intense in the first hour of seizure before diminishing gradually over the next 3 hours. After 2 - 3 hours of continuous seizure activity, convulsive behavioural manifestations become progressively less marked with progression of status epileticus, as observed with clinical status epilepticus [4]. Eventually, the initial overt and violent displays of motor convulsions would be reduced to just rhythmic head-bobbing actions and "blank- stare" appearance as flaccid paralysis sets in and the animals laid sprawl on the floor of their cage [5]. By 24h, all signs of motor convulsions would have largely disappeared [8].

Both human poisoning cases and animal studies have indicated that profound neuropathology and long-term behavioural deficits would ensue if seizures are not controlled promptly [9-13]. From published animal studies, seizures that were not terminated or progressed for at least 40 min produced severe neuropathology and long-term behavioural deficits in all poisoned animals [9-12]. The neuropathology reported includes severe tissue necrosis, neuronal loss, pyknosis and gliosis especially prominent in the piriform and entorhinal cortices, dorsal endopiriform nucleus and the laterodorsal thalamic nucleus. This pattern of injury resembles those described for clinical status epilepticus [4, 12, 14]. In our Soman model, failure to terminate seizure was similarly observed to result in considerable neuronal loss in layers II and III of the piriform cortex (Fig. **2**) and in hilus polymorphic cells within the hippocampus (Fig. **3**) [15].

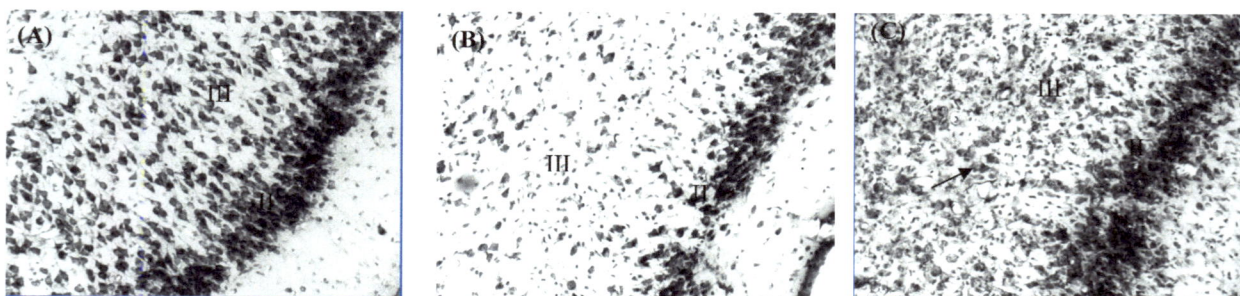

Figure 2: Cellular pathology in piriform cortex of untreated control (A), 1 day post-Soman (C), 1 week post-Soman (E) animal. (Cresyl Violet, x100). Note massive neuronal degeneration at layers II and III highlighted by arrow.

These animal studies reiterated a strong relationship between control of seizures and protection against the lethal effects of nerve agent exposure [11, 16-17]. Hence, as with clinical status epilepticus where rapid seizures control is advocated to minimize the risk of systemic complications [18], early seizures termination during nerve agent poisoning is essential to avoid neuropathology and enhance survival outcomes [11,16-17]. Considering the rapidity in which seizure develops following nerve agent poisoning and its synergistic enhancement of nerve agents' toxicity, concomitant therapeutic administration of anticonvulsant with atropine sulfate and oxime reactivator have been adopted by most military since the early nineties and anticonvulsant is no longer considered as adjunct field therapy [19]. However, for nerve agent-induced seizures, the prognosis of successful neuroprotection is complicated by its underlying aetiology and thus dependent on successful resuscitation efforts to prevent concomitant challenges of cardiopulmonary failure, hypoxia and autonomic complications. These challenges will be elaborated in the following sections.

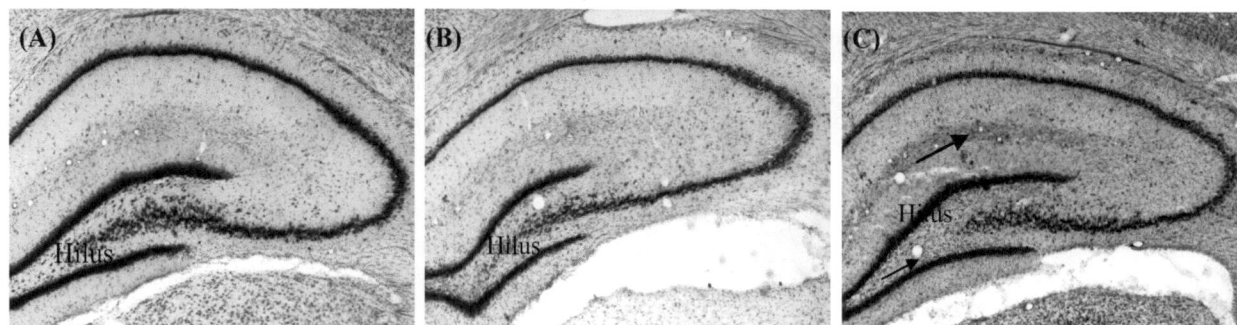

Figure 3: Cellular pathology in hippocampus hilus dentate region of untreated control (A) 1 day post-Soman (B), 1 week post-Soman (C). (Cresyl violet, x100). Note gradual loss of hilus polymorphic cells in (B) and extensive gliosis highlighted by arrows in (C).

CURRENT UNDERSTANDING ON AETIOLOGY OF NERVE AGENT-INDUCED SEIZURES

Status epilepticus initiated by nerve agent poisoning evolved through the same 5 phases of electrocorticographic (EEG) changes as observed in alternate animal models of generalised convulsive seizures (*i.e.*, kainic acid, bicuculline and lithium/pilocarpine). This reflects a common underlying neurochemical mechanism in the initiation and maintenance of status epilepticus [5, 13, 20-21]. The similarities between convulsive status in rodent and human have been previously demonstrated by Treiman and co-workers [22], which forms the basis for extrapolating animal observations of nerve agent-induced seizures in animal as prognostic outcomes of nerve agent-seizures in human.

In terms of neurochemical changes, nerve agent induced-seizures is hypothesised to occur through two distinct stages, an initial cholinergic phase followed through an intermediate transition phase to an established status epilepticus phase driven by non-cholinergic neurochemistry [16]. Following nerve agent-inhibition of acetylcholinesterase, accumulation of excess acetylcholine in the central nervous system triggers generalised brain hyper-excitability. Evidence for the involvement of a cholinergic phase in seizures initiation came from both observations of enhanced release of acetylcholine shortly before seizure onset and the pronounced ability of anti-cholinergic drugs to either prevent seizures onset or to terminate seizures when administered shortly after seizures onset [23].

This initial cholinergic phase-induced hyper-excitation recruits additional neurotransmitter systems to help propagate the developing seizures. This forms the transition phase that was proposed to commence 5-10 minutes post seizures onset [16]. During this phase of seizures propagation, the involvement of additional neurotransmitter systems results in rapid deterioration in the ability of anti-cholinergic drugs to terminate status epilepticus, reflected as escalation of required drug doses to terminate seizures [24]. After an interval of 30-40 minutes of continuous seizure activity, it enters into the phase of established status epilepticus and its driving neurochemistry takes on a predominantly non-cholinergic nature [16].

While the primary importance of acetylcholine as the driving force in the initial cholinergic phase is largely uncontested, there is greater diversity in scientific opinions on the role various neurotransmitter systems played in the transition and established phases of status epilepticus. Glutamate, gamma amino-butyric acid (GABA), dopamine and norepinephrine neurotransmitter systems have all been cited to exert major influences in the propagation and maintenance of status epilepticus. The relative importance of each neurotransmitter system and efficacy of anticonvulsants targeting these neurotransmitter systems will be discussed in greater details in the following paragraphs.

Glutamatergic System

Glutamate neurochemistry is commonly cited in literature as the driving force for propagating and maintaining the established and refractory phases of status epilepticus in nerve agent poisoned animals [16, 23]. Elevated levels of glutamate will depolarise post-synaptic neurons by binding to non-NMDA receptors such as AMPA and metabotrophic glutamate receptor subtype 5 (mGluR5). The resultant excessive depolarisation induced by AMPA and mGluR5 receptors would remove the magnesium ion blockade of NMDARs, thus generating the NMDAR current that sustains status epilepticus. Excessive release of glutamate from excited neurons will continue during recurrent, prolonged or intense seizures, resulting in a vicious self-perpetuating cycle [7, 16, 23].

The role of glutamate in sustaining established status epilepticus is validated by the use of NMDA receptor antagonists, which were found to be effective in terminating established status epileticus in experimental animals [8, 25-26]. Excessive activation of NMDA receptor would in turn lead to accumulation of intracellular calcium, activation of various proteases and eventual neuronal death [7].

Much of current research for alternate neuroprotectant drugs is centred on NMDA receptor antagonist compounds. While current generation of NMDA drugs exhibit neuroprotective effects during established status, they have several critical drawbacks that rendered human applications non-viable. These drawbacks include potent psychomimetic properties leading to hyper-reactive behaviour and memory impairment. They are also determined to have narrow therapeutic window, being neurotoxic at high doses by facilitating apoptotic death in healthy neurons [27-28]. Hence, despite two decades of research on NMDA receptor antagonists, none is yet approved for clinical application.

A new generation of non-competitive NMDA antagonist drugs is being evaluated as neuroprotectants against nerve agent-induced status epilepticus. These included GK-11 or Gascyclidine, a non-competitive NMDA receptor antagonist [29] and HU-211, a dexanabinol that acts as a functional antagonist of the NMDA receptor but which lacks cannabimimetic activity [30]. Both are currently in early phases of clinical trials and neither has been approved for human application till date.

GABAergic System

Gamma aminobutyric acid receptors (GABARs) are heteromeric protein complexes composed of multiple subunits that form ligand-gated anion-selective channels that are modulated by barbiturates, benzodiazepines, ethanol, volatile anesthetics and the anesthetic steroids. Activation of post-synaptic $GABA_A$ receptors by GABA results in synaptic inhibition in the forebrain to depress central nervous system (CNS) hyper-excitability induced by acetylcholine and glutamate neurotransmitters. Imbalance in CNS levels of excitatory and inhibitory neurotransmitters will tilt towards seizures initiation [31].

With prolonged seizures (20-40 minutes), $GABA_A$ receptor-mediated inhibition in the dentate gyrus would be reduced. The loss of GABAR-mediated inhibition is attributed to increased expression of the α-4 subunit in the GABA receptor protein following prolonged status epilepticus. The conformation change results in the loss of affinity and activity of the receptor to GABA actions [7, 32]. As the dentate gyrus normally acts to restrict the flow of epileptiform activity into the hippocampus and hence retard the development of generalised seizures, reducing the GABAR-inhibitory control would lead to maximal activation of the hippocampus and dentate gyrus.

Once the hippocampal-parahippocampal loop is activated, the dentate gyrus sustains self-reinforcing seizures and from this initial focal reverberating circuit, seizures spread to other limbic structures as well as cortical forebrain areas [33]. Once generalised seizures set in, the reverberating circuits enlarge to encompass a cortico-subcorticol nature. This enlarged pacemaker circuit is self-reinforcing and acts, through a combination of breakdown of endogenous inhibitory mechanisms and enhancement of excitatory pathways, to perpetuate seizure discharges. Hence, loss of GABA mediated inhibitory synaptic transmission in the hippocampus is suggested to be critical for the emergence of status epilepticus [34].

The anticonvulsant fielded by most countries for managing nerve agent induced seizures is diazepam, a benzodiazepine that targets $GABA_A$ receptors to enhance $GABA_A$-mediated inhibition of neuronal excitability [31]. Diazepam bioavailability following intramuscular administration is reported to be erratic, with C_{max} reached after 95 minutes in healthy volunteers and between 1- 24 h in adult patients [35-36]. However, once it enters the systemic circulation, being a highly lipophilic compound, diazepam enters the brain quickly to exert its anticonvulsant action. Unfortunately, being highly lipophilic, it also quickly redistributes and it has been shown in an animal model that the highest concentration of diazepam in the brain occurred immediately after intravenous infusion before falling off rapidly, paralleling the rapid decline in plasma concentration [37- 38].

In man, after an intravenous dose of 0.3 mg/kg, plasma concentration reportedly fell below 200 µg/l within 50 minutes, with the latter concentration being considered as the minimum plasma concentration required for suppressing status epilepticus in human [39]. As a result, seizures may recur and this transient anticonvulsant effect of diazepam (< 2 h) is noted in nerve agent poisoned animals [37, 40]. This is in agreement with clinical findings of transient efficacy with diazepam in controlling conventional status epilepticus as well as with the recurrence of seizures after initial successful seizures termination [39, 41-42]. In view of its inconsistent absorption from the intramuscular site and inability to rapidly achieve sufficient therapeutic doses for terminating seizures, most clinicians have consistently advised against intramuscular administration for diazepam in the field.

The other commonly applied anticonvulsant in clinical practice is lorazepam. Like diazepam, it manifests anticonvulsant activity within minutes of absorption but is reported to have a better safety profile in children [43]. However, in animal models, lorazepam is less effective than diazepam in arresting nerve agent-induced seizures. Moreover, like diazepam, lorazepam is a highly lipophilic compound and hence not an optimal choice when intravenous access is not available since it has a similar variable absorption after intramuscular administration.

In recent publications, studies with midazolam have advocated this compound as a more effective benzodiazepine for arresting nerve agent induced seizures when administered intramuscularly [17, 44-47]. Although many experts in chemical defense increasingly favor midazolam, it should also be noted that midazolam has a short circulation half-life and faces the same challenge as diazepam with seizures recurrence after initial successful seizure termination [48-49].

Benzodiazepines as a class of anticonvulsant faced another major limitation when administered late post seizure onset. With prolonged status, conformation changes in $GABA_A$ receptor is reported to result in increased pharmacoresistance to benzodiazepines & barbiturate, resulting in reduced anticonvulsant effects in both animals and human subjects [7, 50-51] Hence, while diazepam could arrest seizures when applied within 5 min of seizure onset, its anticonvulsant efficacy drops rapidly with further delays in administration. When administered 40 minutes post-seizure onset, diazepam has limited anticonvulsant efficacy in nerve agent poisoned animals [52]. Increasing diazepam dose to circumvent this developing pharmaco-resistance in the field is potentially dangerous due to benzodiazepines ability to potentiate nerve agent-induced respiratory depression. Unfortunately, non-arrested status epilepticus in nerve agent casualties would have become refractory by the time these casualties reached the hospitals. Hence, it is often vital for seizures to be arrested in the field.

Within hospitals intensive care wards, anaesthesia-induced coma is effective for seizures suppression when dealing with refractory status epileptics [18]. Nonetheless, this does not prevent neuropathology initiated by the earlier events of status epilepticus prior to coma induction [53]. In fact, even when seizure is terminated 20 minutes post seizures onset, mild neuropathology was already evident in the treated animals [11, 16-17]. From our own experiments, we observed that diazepam, even when used at a supra-high dose of 10 mg/kg, was unable to terminate all cases of seizure even when administered 30 minutes post seizure onset. Similar findings, with an even higher dose of 20 mg/kg diazepam, were reported by Filbert's team [54]. Hence, serious concerns remain on the ability of the current diazepam based autoinjector device to deal with nerve agent seizures, particularly when it is used on casualties with established status epilepticus in the field.

Dopaminergic System

In a series of studies conducted initially by Fosbraey [55] and followed up by Jacobsson and Cassel [56-57], Soman-induced seizures was reported to result in delayed (>40 min following seizure onset) increases in extracellular dopamine levels in the brain. With moderate soman intoxication, beside increased GABA release, enhanced release in dopamine was the only other significant neurochemical change in the striatum area. These studies also correlated animals exhibiting marked signs of poisoning with enhanced CNS release of dopamine. As oxidative deamination of dopamine32 will result in the formation of free radicals in the brain, massive release of dopamine was suggested to generate oxidative stress on striatal neurons, leading to increased neuronal loss in the striatum region. However, in view of the delayed nature of the increase in dopamine efflux, it is likely that dopamine neurochemistry is relatively less important in the initial propagation of nerve agent seizures [16].

Noradrenergic System

Nerve agent inhibition of synaptic acetylcholinesterase results in sustained excitation of pre-synaptic nicotinic receptors of norepinephrine-containing neurons located at the locus coeruleus (LC). This results in sustained secondary release of norepinephrine (NE) from the LC terminals. Hence, a convulsive dose of nerve agent will result in excessive releases of both acetylcholine (ACh) and NE in the central nervous system, elevating extracellular concentrations of both neurotransmitters [58]. Statistically significant reductions in neuronal NE content were observed in all brain regions 5-10 minutes after the onset of nerve agent-induced seizure activity. NE levels in the brain proceeded to decline to 20-30% of normal level over the next few hours of intoxication [59].

Besides attributing the depletion in neuronal NE store to cholinergic-induced neuronal excitation, disruption of NE recovery within the central nervous system during status epilepticus was proposed by the authors to be another important factor in its depletion. NE action is terminated *in vivo* by re-uptake mechanisms into noradrenergic nerve terminals. There are two such innate mechanisms, uptake 1 and uptake 2, corresponding to neuronal and extra-neuronal uptake respectively [60]. Uptake 1 mechanism belongs to a family of neurotransmitter proteins, which act as co-transporters of sodium and chloride ions and the amine in question. Uptake 1 co-transporters rely on the sodium electrochemical gradient as a driving force for recovery of NE into the terminal cytosol. Changes to this gradient would alter or even reverse the operation of uptake 1 resulting in marked effects on the availability of the released transmitter at post-synaptic receptors.

During nerve agent-induced status epilepticus, profound disruption of this sodium electrochemical gradient is expected. Consequently, re-uptake of NE is likely to occur predominantly through extra-neuronal means, where they are metabolised and not regenerated. This would lead to eventual depletion of NE content *in vivo*. Some authors have postulated this released pool of excess extracellular NE to exert an innate anticonvulsant role in epileptic animal models, mediated through post-synaptic α_2-noradrenergic heteroreceptors, which are located on pre-synaptic nerve fibers [61-63]. Activation of these receptors will inhibit the release of ACh and other non-noradrenergic neurotransmitters [64]. Noradrenergic neurons send these fibres projections into all parts of the forebrain to exert a global control on neuronal excitability. The observed coincidence of seizures onset with rapid depletion of NE content in the brain was thus interpreted by these authors as leading to depletion beyond a critical level of NE inhibitory influence to permit seizures initiation.

However, some *in vitro* studies have also indicated a pro-convulsive role for NE through post-synaptic β-receptors, which may either lower seizure threshold or exacerbate on-going seizure activities [64-66]. Reports of anticonvulsant actions of propranolol, a post-synaptic β-receptor antagonist, against pentylenetetrazol-induced convulsions in rats [65] supported the contention of NE-mediated seizurogenic mechanism in the early phase of status epilepticus. The absence of NE depletion in nerve agent poisoned animals that did not convulse supported a pro-convulsive role for NE during the initial propagation phase of nerve agent seizures [59]. These assertions were also supported by reports of successful termination of maximal electroshock-induced seizures by β-adrenergic drugs [65-66]. However, with Soman-poisoned animals, these drugs were less effective in seizures arrest [67].

Prophylactic application of α_2-noradrenergic receptor agonist drugs, such as clonidine, has been demonstrated in the eighties [67-70] to prevent Soman-induced convulsions and dose-related inhibition of Soman-induced cardio-vascular deficits (Fig. 4) [71-72]. This compound acts on both pre-synaptic and postsynaptic α_2-adrenergic receptors on both cholinergic as well as locus coeruleus (LC) neurons to inhibit the release of acetylcholine (ACh) and norepinephrine (NE) respectively.

However, subsequent studies by Shih and co-workers indicated that clonidine's anticonvulsant actions, when applied as a pretreatment, was restricted to a narrow dose range [52]. At higher doses, besides the absence of anticonvulsant effects, prophylactic applications of clonidine were constantly accompanied by pronounced behavioral and EEG effects. Further doubts on the importance of noradrenergic system in nerve agent seizures propagation were raised with reports demonstrating feasibility of initiating status epilepticus by microinjection of nerve agents into discrete brain regions distant from the locus coeruleus neurons [58]. Such data, however, should not be used to discount the contribution of norepinephrine system towards the propagation and maintenance of nerve agent seizures. This is in view of the known ability of discrete seizures, generated by microinjections, to spread to other parts of the brain such as the locus coeruleus neurons to induce the release of excessive amounts of NE.

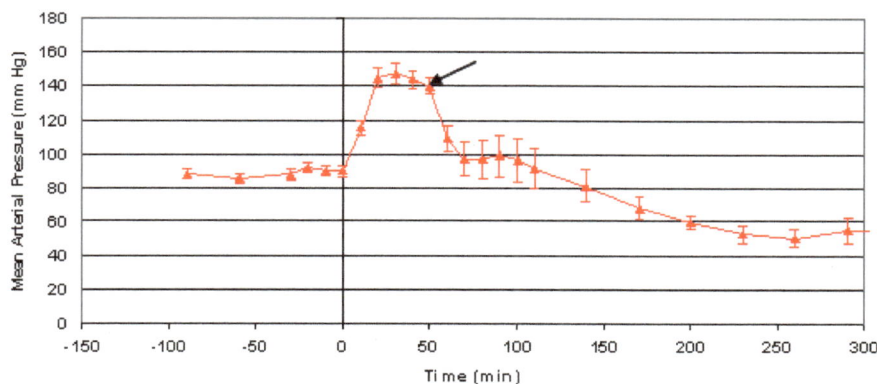

Figure 4: Changes in Mean arterial blood pressure following Soman. Post-treatment with Clonidine (2mg/kg) and 64 mg/kg atropine (C), (arrow) reverses Soman pressor effect.

The apparent dual, pro-convulsant and anti-convulsant, roles of NE is related to the receptor type that is stimulated. There are 4 types of adrenergic receptors in the central nervous system, namely α_1, α_2, β_1, β_2. Each of the α_1- and α_2-receptors each have 3 different receptor subtypes: α_{1A}-, α_{1B}-, α_{1D}-. α_{2A}-, α_{2A}-, α_{2c}- subtype. NE excitatory response is mediated through β-receptors and/or α_1- receptors while its inhibitory effects are mediated through α_2-receptors [73]. These receptors are distributed in different pre- and pro-synaptic locations and NE can exert either pro-convulsive or anti-convulsive effects depending on its site of release and eventual action [74].

During progression of status epilepticus in nerve agent poisoned animals, the initial amount of NE released from stimulation of LC neurons gradually collates into a huge flood of synaptic NE levels, which flows into the surrounding areas around the synapses, stimulating all different types of adrenergic receptors. This may account for the different interpretations from different research groups of anti-convulsant and pro-convulsant effects of NE.

Most pharmacological agents that target adrenoreceptors, while able to differentiate between the 4 major types of adrenergic receptors, have limited specificity for the receptor subtypes. The common α_2-agonist anticonvulsant studied in the past, clonidine, is non-selective for all 3 α_2-subtypes. As α_{2A}- adrenergic receptors are located both pre-synaptically and post-synaptically, activation of pre-synaptic α_{2A} receptors would inhibit the release of NE to exert pro-convulsant effect. Conversely, activation of the post-synaptic α_{2A} receptors by clonidine would induce anti-convulsant effects by inhibiting the release of acetylcholine.

It is possible that differentiate activation of pre- and post-synaptic α_{2A} receptors is dependent on the extracellular level of clonidine and NE in the CNS. High doses of clonidine administered would result in excessive extracellular concentrations and hence non-discriminative excitation of α_1-adrenergic receptors located pre- and post-synaptically. This may account for the variable protection with clonidine pretreatment and the narrow dose range at which its protective actions were observed [52]. It may also account for the reported behavioural and EEG abnormalities at higher doses of clonidine. Similarly, the abundance of extracellular NE following seizures onset activating all adreno-receptors would mask clonidine anti-convulsant effects mediated through post-synaptic α_{2A} receptors. This could have explained for the distinct lack of anticonvulsant effects when clonidine is applied therapeutically.

THERAPEUTIC EFFECTS OF CLONIDINE-ATROPINE DRUG COMBINATION

Early Application Post Seizures Onset

Prophylactic studies with clonidine in Buccafuso's laboratory revealed synergistic anticonvulsant interactions when it is used in combination with atropine sulfate against Soman poisoning [68]. Atropine sulfate on its own, while being used primarily to attenuate hyper-cholinergic toxicity and restore respiratory sufficiency during nerve agent poisoning, is also reported to prevent seizures when applied prophylactically prior nerve agent administration [52]. However, much higher atropine doses are required to achieve anticonvulsant effects when it was applied early post seizures onset [24, 44, 52].

In our study [6], the effective dose (ED_{50}) dose for atropine to terminate Soman-induced seizure, when applied at 5 minutes post seizures onset, was reduced significantly from 60.32 mg/kg to 8.35 mg/kg (Fig. **5**) with co-administration of clonidine (1 mg/kg; i.m.).

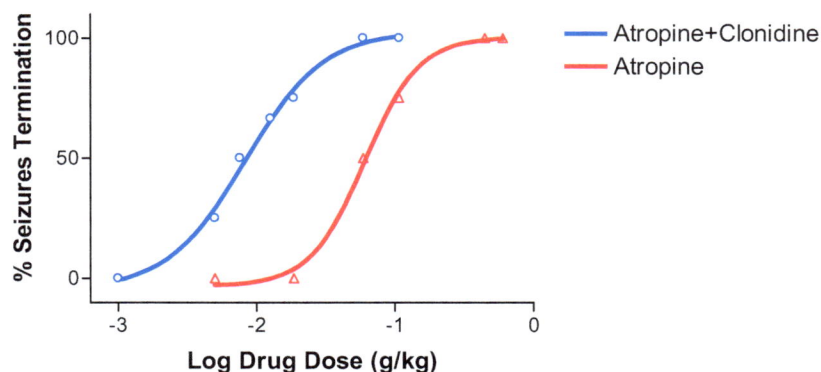

Drug Combination	Atropine	Atropine + Clonidine
ED_{50} (mg/kg, IM)	60.32	8.35
95% Confidence Limits	41.2 – 88.3	5.81 – 12.0

Anticonvulsant Drug Administered 5 min after Soman-Induced seizure onset

Figure 5: Synergistic anticonvulsant effects in a Soman animal from combination of atropine with clonidine

Since clonidine on its own is unable to exert anticonvulsant effects when applied post seizure onset in Soman poisoned animals [52], the significant reduction in atropine's seizures termination dose suggests the existence of a synergistic interaction between clonidine and atropine. Successful anti-convulsant actions of atropine with clonidine drug combinations supported the contention that NE could exert an innate anticonvulsant role through post-synaptic α_2-adrenergic receptors.

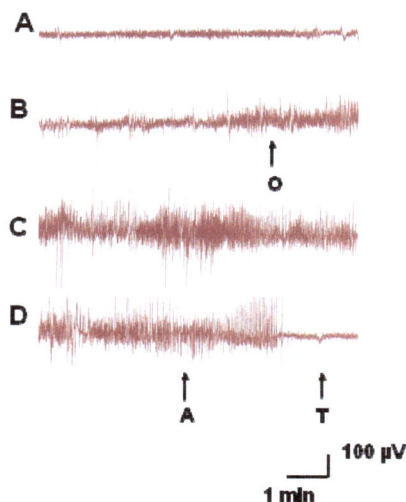

Figure 6: Seizures Terminated Abruptly by Combination of Atropine (107.5 mg/kg) + Clonidine (1 mg/kg)

Seizure termination with this drug combination was remarkably rapid with burst arrest achieved within 2.91 minutes. This compared favourably with 9.62 minutes required using atropine alone (Fig. **6**). This burst arrest rate is superior to that achieved with intramuscularly administered diazepam, which required a mean time of about 50 minutes to achieve burst arrest. It is comparable to midazolam [45, 47], the next generation of benzodiazepine anticonvulsant to be fielded by NATO forces. The absence of respiratory depression with atropine-clonidine anticonvulsant combinations is a comparative advantage to benzodiazepines-based anticonvulsant drugs, which depresses respiration in nerve agent poisoned animals.

Late Application Post Seizures Onset

When administrated late (*i.e.* 40 minutes) post seizure onset, atropine displayed no anticonvulsant properties [24, 44, 52]. Similarly, with tertiary anti-cholinergics compounds such as scopolamine or procyclidine, their anticonvulsant effectiveness are also drastically reduced with delayed administration post seizure onset. Despite its inability to terminate seizures, studies carried out in the author's laboratory [15] indicated that high doses of atropine (128 mg/kg) were surprisingly able to significantly prevent neuronal loss in the piriform cortex compared with untreated Soman controls.

Unfortunately, high doses (128 mg/kg) of atropine administered into Soman-poisoned and hypoxic animals could induce premature ventricular contractions (PVC; Fig. **7**), which developed eventually into ventricular tachycardia and ventricular fibrillation, with death following shortly [15, 75]. This would contra-indicate their application as a neuroprotectant in nerve agent poisoned casualties with established status epilepticus since these casualties are likely to be in hypoxic condition.

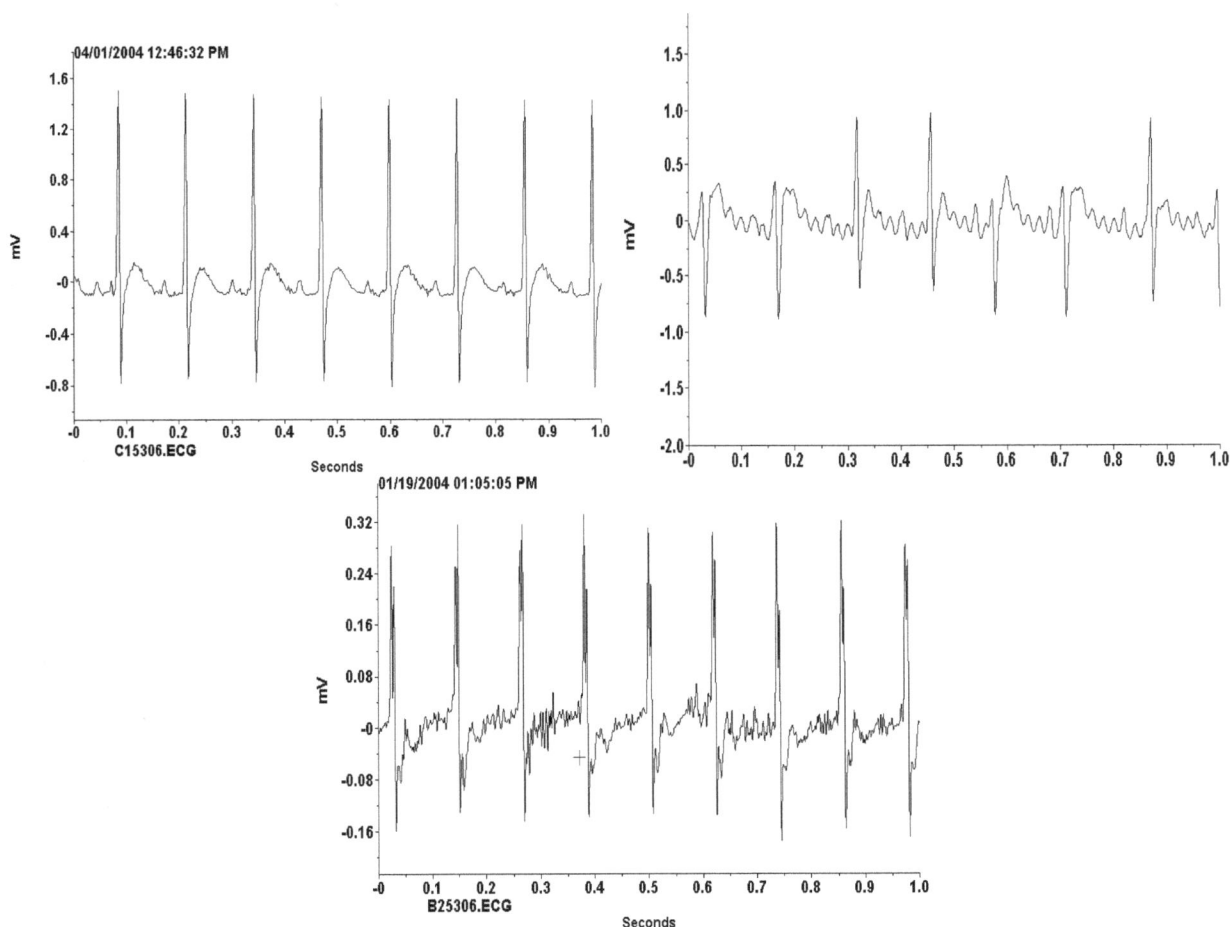

Figure 7: ECG profile of HI-6 pretreated, Soman-poisoned (1.6xLD50) rats with (a) idioventricular rhythm 25-30 minutes post-soman challenge (b) isolated premature ventricular contractions developed after atropine (128 mg/kg) administration at 40 min post seizure onset and (c) normal sinus rhythm restored 10 min after administration of clonidine (2 mg/kg) and atropine (128 mg/kg)

When clonidine was co-administered with atropine in various dose combinations at 40 minutes post seizure onset, seizure arrest was not observed, with the majority of the animals displaying 24 hours of non-stop status epilepticus [75]. This indicates the combined use of clonidine and atropine was also not effective as an anticonvulsant when administered in Soman poisoned animals with established status epilepticus (40 min post seizure onset). However, despite its failure to terminate seizures when administered 40 minutes post-seizure onset, a clonidine-atropine drug combination enhanced atropine neuroprotective effects in the hippocampus (Fig. **8**) and piriform cortex (Fig. **9**). In addition, clonidine co-administration protected the animal against atropine induced ventricular arrhythmias in hypoxic animals (Fig. **7**). Consequently, a clonidine-atropine drug combination was able to significantly enhance the survival rates of Soman poisoned animals beyond that afforded by either drugs alone (Fig. **10**).

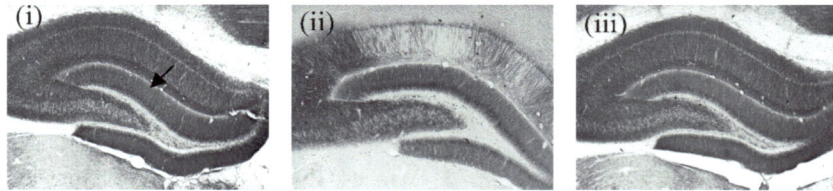

Figure 8: Sections (10 μm) of hippocampus from a (i) normal animal, (ii) Soman poisoned animal (176ug/kg), arrows indicated region with loss of microtubule -associated protein (MAP), a marker of seizure-related brain damage[76](iii) Soman poisoned animal given clonidine 2 mg/kg and atropine 8 mg/kg 40 minutes post seizure onset (MAP2 immuno -staining, x40).

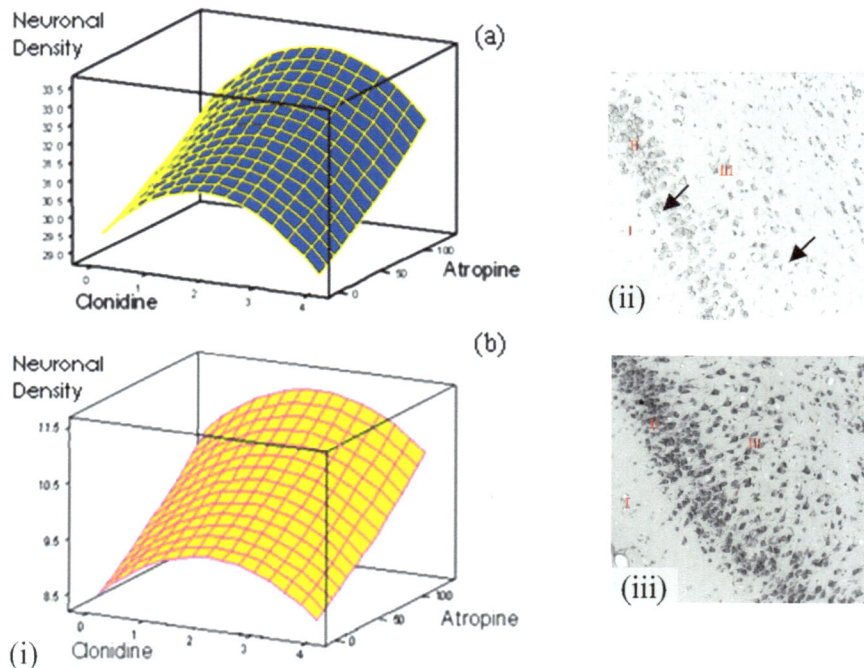

Figure 9: (i) 3-D representations of neuronal density in layers II (a) and III (c) of the piriform cortex as a function of atropine sulfate and clonidine doses. Neuronal density is defined as the ratio of area covered by neurons to the total brain area observed under the microscope; (ii) 10 μm sections of piriform cortex from a Soman (1.6xLD$_{50}$) poisoned animal, with regions of neuron loss indicated (arrows) and from (iii) a Soman poisoned animal given clonidine 2 mg/kg and atropine 8 mg/kg 40 minutes after onset of seizure (Cresyl Violet, x100).

The feasibility to prevent neuropathology in the absence of seizures arrest was also reported in a separate study with a combination of diazepam and dantrolene administered to a Soman poisoned animal at a state of established status epilepticus [54]. In that study, Filbert and her co-workers demonstrated significant neuroprotection could be achieved in all brain regions with the application of a supra-high dose of diazepam (20 mg/kg), with and without co-administered dantrolene. This neuroprotective effect was achieved despite the continued presence of seizures and status epilepticus. Filbert's team thus concluded that diazepam, alone or in combination with dantrolene, offers promise as a viable neuroprotection regimen in casualties with established status epilepticus.

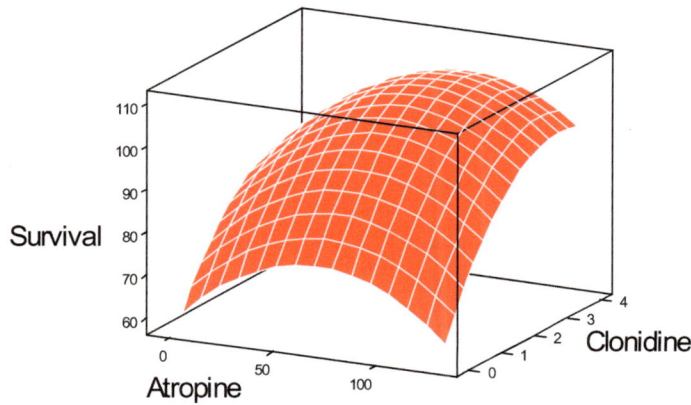

Figure 10: Survival rate of Soman poisoned animals treated with various combinations of atropine sulphate and clonidine at 40 min post seizure onset (n=6 animals per drug dose combination).

A comparative study was thus undertaken to compare the overall protection and neuroprotection afforded by diazepam and atropine sulphate as compared with an optimal clonidine (2 mg/kg) - atropine (64 mg/kg) drug combination. The optimal dosages were predicted from experimental data using response surface modelling module in Minitab (ver. 13). The 0.4 mg/kg diazepam dose chosen approximated the current total dose obtained from three diazepam autoinjectors (10 mg per autoinjector) given to a 75-kg human.

Soman-controls (GD) have the lowest survival rates at 38% (Fig. **11**). Animals that received the additional combinatory treatment of clonidine (2 mg/kg) and atropine sulfate (64 mg/kg; C2AS64) 40 minutes post seizure onset recorded the highest 24h survival rate of 79% [15]. Delaying this drug combination administration to 70 min post seizures onset did not reduce its protective effects. In comparison, much lower survival rates of 51% and 46% were observed respectively in animals that received diazepam (0.4 mg/kg) with atropine (0.2 mg/kg; D0.4AS0.2) or diazepam (0.4 mg/kg; D0.4) alone. Adding diazepam (0.4 mg/kg) to the clonidine with atropine combination (C2AS64D0.4) did not further enhance the 24h survival rate (78%) of Soman-poisoned animals.

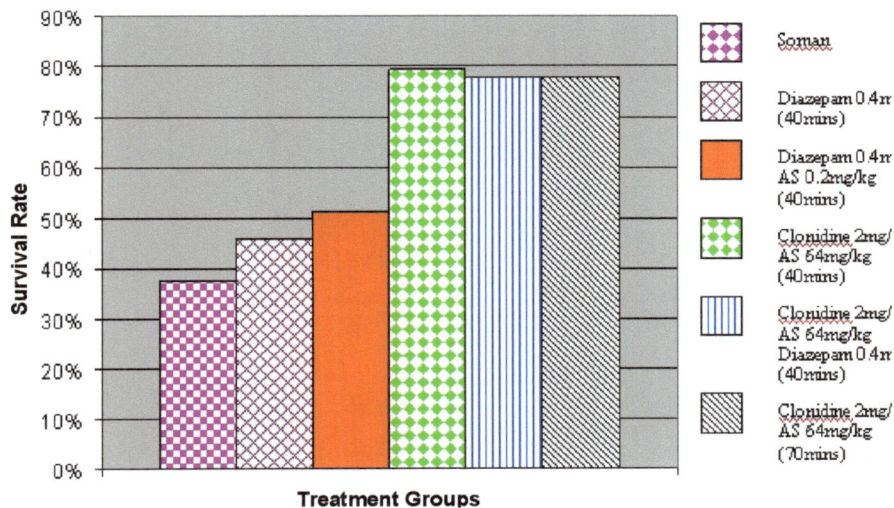

Figure 11: Survival rates amongst Soman poisoned animals treated with clonidine-atropine sulphate, diazepam, diazepam-atropine and clonidine-atropine-diazepam combinations. Clonidine-atropine combination was given at either 40 or 70 min post seizure onset.

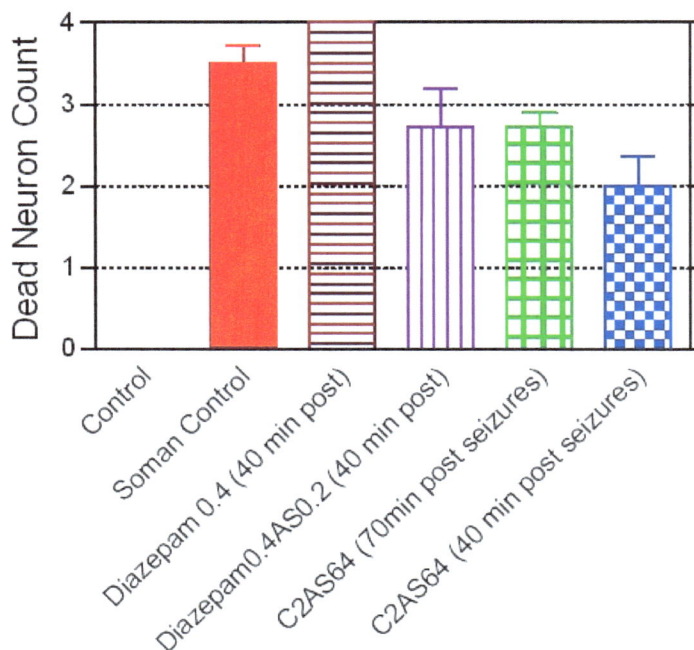

Figure 12: Score of degenerating neurons stained by fluoro jade in layer II of the piriform cortex on Day 8 following Soman intoxication and post seizure (40 min) treatments. Score as "0 - No dying cells; 1 - <20 dying cells; 2 - between 20 to 50 cells; 3 - >50 dying cells and 4 - Obvious tissue damage/disintegrated".

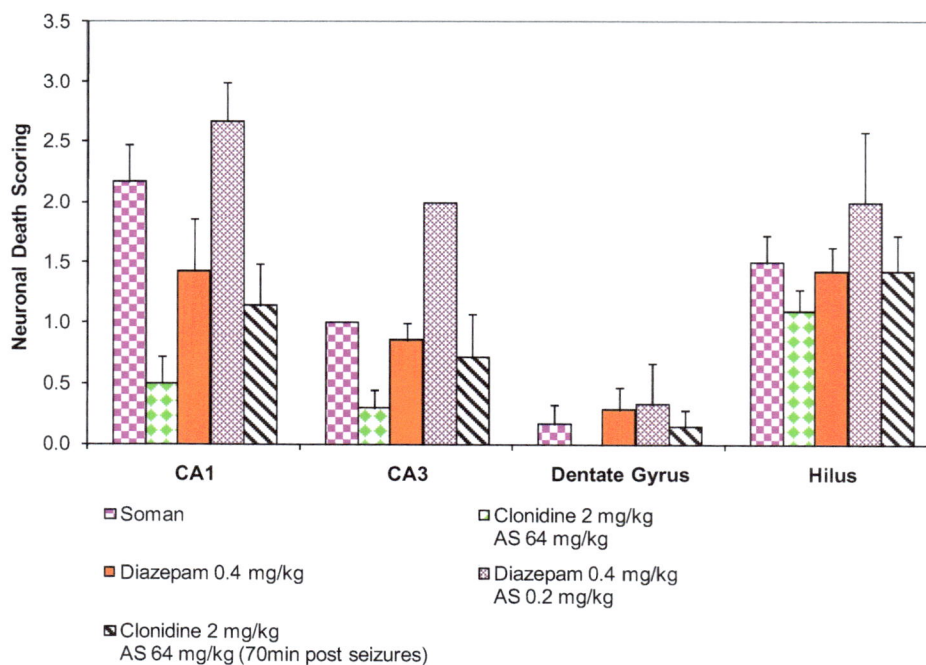

Figure 13: Score of degenerating neurons stained by fluoro jade in different regions of the hippocampus on Day 8 following Soman intoxication and post seizure (40 min) treatments. Score as "0 - No dying cells; 1 - <20 dying cells; 2 - between 20 to 50 cells; 3 - >50 dying cells and 4 - Obvious tissue damage/disintegrated".

The neuropathology in these animals were determined using fluoro jade staining [77], which selectively stains for degenerating neuronal cells. Diazepam alone, when given at 40 min post seizures onset, did not reduce neuropathology in the piriform cortex (Fig. **12**) as assessed from brain sections obtained from animals euthanized 8 days post Soman poisoning. Addition of atropine sulfate to diazepam reduced neuropathology while the neuroprotective combination of clonidine and atropine significantly reduced the numbers of dead neurons by 50%. Delaying the clonidine-atropine treatment to 70 min post seizure onset increased the dead neuron score by 1 unit (Fig. **13**). Similar findings were observed across all the regions in the hippocampus with the highest amount of neuronal death observed with the Soman controls.

Diazepam-treated animals demonstrated minimal neuronal protection as opposed to animals that received the clonidine-atropine combination at 40 min post seizures, which had the lowest level of neuronal death. Delaying the clonidine-atropine treatment to 70 min post seizure onset was also observed to increase the number of dead neurons in all regions of the hippocampus. As the hippocampus is an integral structure involved in learning and memory functions of the brain, concomitant with the observed loss of neurons in Soman poisoned animals, the cognitive ability of these animals were drastically reduced 8 days post intoxication when evaluated using Morris Water Maze tests (Fig. **14**). On the other hand, animals treated at 40 min post-seizure onset with the clonidine-atropine drug combination provided far superior cognitive performance as compared to both the

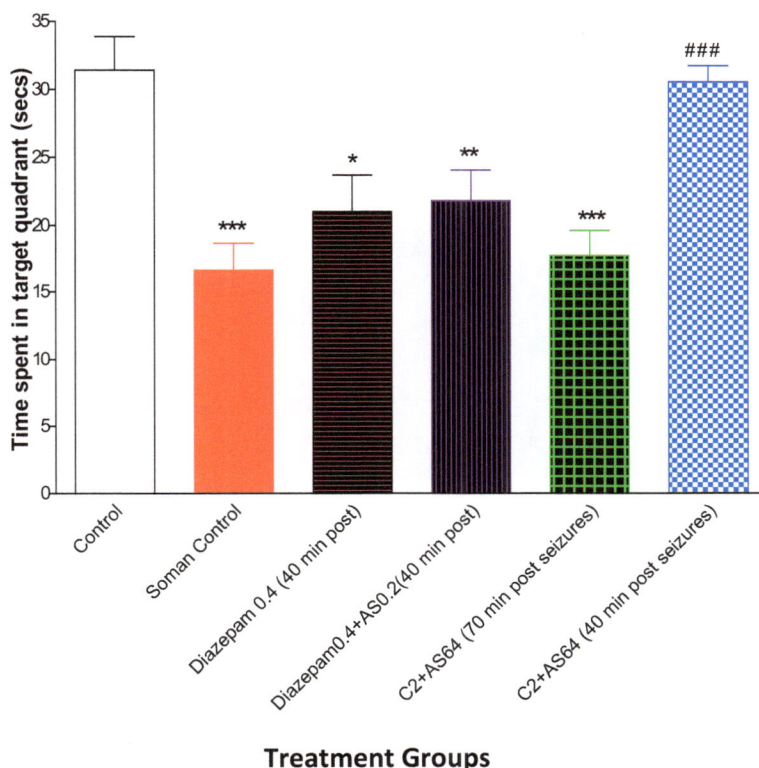

Treatment Groups

Figure 14: Morris maze memory test results of Soman-intoxicated animals (with and without post-treatments) as reflected by the time spent in the target quadrant at Day 8 post soman challenge. Significant differences (t- tests) against control indicated as * ($p<0.1$), ** ($p<0.01$) and *** ($p<0.001$) while significance against Soman indicated by [###] ($p<0.001$)

Soman poisoned animals that did not receive any neuroprotectant treatment or Soman-poisoned animals post-treated with diazepam (with or without co-administered atropine sulfate). Interesting, the cognitive performance of animals post treated with clonidine and atropine at 40 min post seizure onset was found to be similar to those of normal animals who were not poisoned by Soman [15]. However, when the clonidine-atropine treatment was delayed to 70 min post seizure onset, cognitive performance deteriorated significantly and was equivalent to Soman poisoned animals.

To understand how clonidine assisted in enhancing atropine neuroprotective effects, microdialysis studies were carried out to determine the extracellular level of acetylcholine in the brain following Soman poisoning and administration of this neuroprotective drug combination at 40 min post seizure onset. From the data gathered (Fig. 15), administration of a high dose of atropine (8 mg/kg) resulted in a late surge in acetylcholine efflux. Hence, while a high level of atropine is required to block over-excitation at the post-synaptic muscarinic receptors, such high atropine levels could also act on pre-synaptic muscarinic M_2 receptors to block innate feedback mechanisms resulting in continuous release of acetylcholine from the pre-synaptic junction and perpetuating the neurotoxic effects of Soman poisoning.

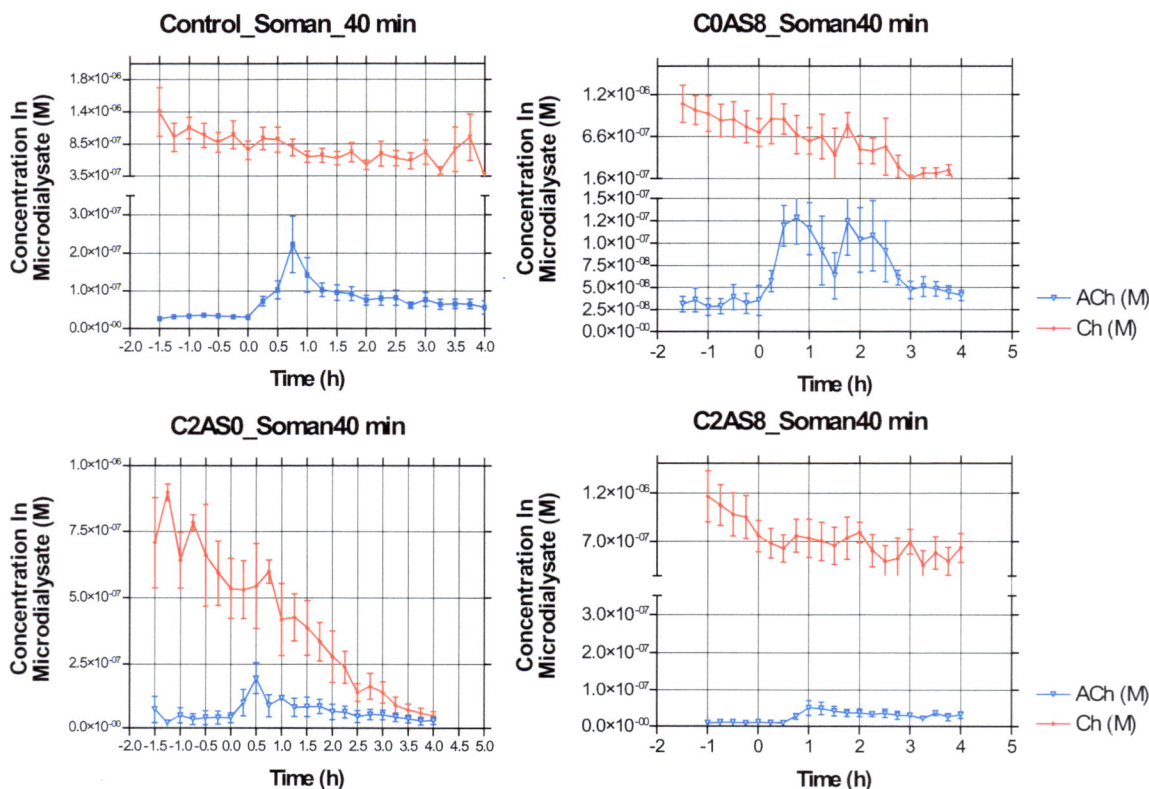

Figure 15: Changes in Extracellular Concentration of Acetylcholine and Choline in Basal Ganglia of Soman Poisoned Rats (1.6 x LD50; s.c.) with and without co-administration of clonidine (C2; 2 mg/kg) and atropine (AS8; 8mg/kg), at 40 minutes post-seizure onset. (n=6 animals per dose combination).

Clonidine acting on post-synaptic α_{2A}-noradrenergic receptors, located on cholinergic neurons receiving noradrenergic innervation [73], was observed to reduce acetylcholine efflux even when applied 40 min post seizure onset. When used as a clonidine-atropine combination treatment, the level of acetylcholine outflow was further curtailed to near basal levels. Combined with atropine blocking post-synaptic activation of muscarinc receptors, this treatment combination would dampen excitatory inputs from the cholinergic system. Without atropine post-synaptic blockage actions, pre-synaptic control of acetylcholine release by clonidine alone would have limited influences on the spread of neuronal excitation in the brain.

The ability of clonidine-atropine drug combination to provide neuroprotection and the observed reduction of acetylcholine outflow by this drug combination during established status epilepticus challenges current assumption that established status epilepticus phase is driven primarily non-cholinergic neurochemistry [16]. As the underlying aetiology arising from nerve agent involves inhibition of synaptic acetylcholinesterase, the cholinergic system may still play a prominent role in determining the eventual degree of neuropathology in casualties with unabated seizures following nerve agent poisoning.

SUMMARY

This study is perhaps the first successful demonstration of manipulating central α_2-adrenergic and cholinergic receptors for neuroprotective effects in nerve agent poisoned and hypoxic animals with established status epilepticus. The findings suggest that a combination of drugs targeting central muscarinic and adrenergic receptors could be an alternative neuroprotection option to current choice of benzodiazepine drugs that carries significant risks of respiratory depression amongst nerve agent casualties.

The study also provided a new understanding in the search for neuroprotective drugs to treat nerve agent-induced seizure as none of the drugs used in this study has direct antagonistic or modulatory actions on glutamate receptors such as the N-methyl-D-aspartate (NMDA) receptor. Hence, despite current suggestions that countering glutamate excitotoxicity is instrumental in preventing neuropathology amongst nerve agent-poisoned animals, the study outcome points out distinctly that it is possible to achieve neuroprotection without targeting the glutamate system directly through the use of NMDA-specific drugs [78]. It also should renew interests to investigate the role cholinergic systems may play in resultant neuropathology amongst casualties with unabated seizures.

It is important in this study [15] and similar findings from other research groups [54] that significant neuroprotection and animal survival could be achieved despite the inability of such medications to arrest seizures. Hence, it may not be totally accurate to state that termination of seizures to be the over-riding factor influencing the survival rates and neuroprotection amongst nerve agent-intoxicated animals [17]. These may influence the search for alternate neuroprotection drugs and treatment regimes to current diazepam option for managing hypoxic casualties with established status epilepticus.

Finally, the observed inability of this clonidine-atropine drug combination to prevent neuronal loss when applied during the refractory status epilepticus phase (70 min post seizure onset) was similar to findings of limited neuroprotection with ketamine-atropine combination during the refractory phase. These data suggests that more complex neural cascades and neuroinflammatory processes may have been initiated once nerve agent-induced seizures reach the refractory status epilepticus stage. Accumulating data suggests that seizure-induced microglial activation and up-regulation of pro-inflammatory cytokines can lead to neuronal injury [79-81]. A totally different treatment approach may hence be required to manage such casualties to enhance survival and limit brain damage [82].

REFERENCES

[1]   Marrs TC, Maynard RL, Sidell FR, Ed. Organophosphate nerve agents. In: Chemical warfare agents, toxicology and treatment. New York: John Wiley & Sons Ltd. 1996; pp 83-101.

[2]   Somani SM, Solana RP, Dube SN. Toxicodynamics of Nerve Agents In: Somani SM Ed., Chemical warfare agents. San Diego, California: Academic Press Inc. 1992; pp 68-108

[3]   Karalliedde L, Henry JA. Effects of organophosphates on skeletal muscles. Hum Exp Toxicol 1993; 12: 289-296.

[4]   Shorvon S. Chapter 4 -Neurophysiology, neuropathology and neurochemistry of status epilepticus. In: Shorvon S. Ed. Status Epilepticus - Its clinical features and treatment in children and adults; Cambridge University Press. 1992; pp 144-145.

[5]   Irwin Koplovitz, John P. Skvorak. Electrocorticographic changes during generalised convulsive status epilepticus in Soman-intoxicated rats. Epilepsy Res 1998; 30: 159-164.

[6]   Loke WK, Alicia Ho LK, Chua-Soh PC, Tan YT, Ho ML. Anticonvulsant Effects of Post-Intoxication Administered Atropine Clonidine Drug Combination In Soman-Poisoned Rats. In : Proceedings of the 7th International Symposium on Protection Against Chemical and Biological Warfare Agents, Stockholm, Sweden, Jun 14-19, 2001.

[7]   Kapur J, Macdonald RL. Chapter 18 - Status epilepticus: a proposed pathophysiology. In : Shorvon S, Dreifuss F, Fish D and Thomas D, Ed. The treatment of epilepsy. London: Blackwell Science Ltd. 1996; pp 258-268.

[8]   Sparenborg S, Braitman DJ. Dizocilpine (MK-801) arrests status epilepticus and prevents brain damage induced by Soman. Neuropharmacology 1992; 31: 357-368.

[9]   Petras JM. Neurology and neuropathology of Soman-induced brain injury: an overview. JEAB 1994; 61: 319-329

[10]   McDonough JH Jr. Protection against nerve agent-induced neuropathology, but not cardiac pathology, is associated with the anticonvulsant action of drug pretreatment. NeuroToxicology 1995; 15: 123-132

[11]   McDonough JH Jr. Relationship between seizure control and protection against soman-induced lethality in guinea pigs. In: Proceedings of the 1996 Medical Defence Bioscience Review; 1996 May 12-16, Baltimore, USA. Baltimore, USA: USA Army Medical Research and Material Command, 1996.

[12]   Corsellis JAN, Bruton CJ Neuropathology of status epilepticus in humans. In: Delgado-Escueta AV, Wasterlain CG, Treiman DM, Porter RJ Ed. Status epilepticus- mechanisms of brain damage and treatment. Advances in Neurology, Vol 34, New York: Raven Press. 1983; pp 129-139..

[13]   Meldrum BS, Horton RW. Physiology of status epilepticus in primates. Arch Neurol 1973; 28:1-9

[14]   Oxbury JM, Whitty CWM. Causes and consequences of status epilepticus in adults: a study of 86 cases. Brain 1971; 94: 733-744.

[15]   Loke WK, Alicia Ho LK, Loo HK, Chua-Soh PC. Ong BL. Neuroprotection Options for Treatment of Nerve Agent-Induced Status Epilepticus. In: 2nd Singapore International Neuroscience Conference- Mechanisms, Models & Medicine, Singapore, July 22-23, 2004.

[16]   McDonough JH Jr, Shih TM. Neuropharmacological mechanisms of nerve agent-induced seizure and neuropathology. Neurosci Biobehav Rev 1997; 21: 559-579.

[17]   Shih TM, Duniho SM, McDonough JH Jr. Control of nerve agent-induced seizures is critical for neuroprotection and survival. Toxicol Appl Pharmacol. 2003;188: 69-80.

[18]   Shorvon S. Chapter 6 - Prognosis and outcome of status epilepticus. In: Shorvon S. Ed. Status epilepticus - its clinical features and treatment in children and adults. Cambridge University Press. 1992; pp 293-301,

[19]   Dunn MA, Sidell FR. Progress in medical defence against nerve agents. J.A.M.A. 1989; 262: 649-652.

[20]   Ben-Ari Y. Limbic seizure and brain damage produced by kainic acid: mechanisms and relevance to human temporal lobe epilepsy. Neuroscience 1985; 14: 375-403.

[21]   Tang FR, Lee WL, Yang J, Sim MK, Ling EA. Metabotropic glutamate receptor 8 in the rat hippocampus after pilocarpine induced status epilepticus. Neurosci Lett 2000; 286: 1-4.

[22]   Treiman DM. Walton NY, Kendrick CA. Progressive sequence of electroencephalographic changes during generalised convulsive status epilepticus. Epilepsy Res 1990; 5: 49-60.

[23]   Shih TM, McDonough JH Jr. Neurochemical mechanisms in Soman-induced seizures. J Appl Toxicol 1997; 17: 255-264.

[24]   McDonough JH, Jr, Zoeffel LD, McMonagle J, Copeland TL, Smith CD and Shih TM. Anticonvulsant treatment of nerve agent seizures: anticholinergics versus diazepam in Soman-intoxicated guinea pigs. Epilepsy Res 2000; 38: 1-14.

[25]   Carpentier P, Foquin-Tarricone A, Bodjarian N, Rondouin G, Lerner-Natoli M, Kamenka JM, Blanchet G, Denoyer M, Lallement G. Anticonvulsant and antilethal effects of the phencyclidine derivative TCP in soman poisoning. NeuroToxicology 1994; 15: 837-852.

[26]   Lallement G, Clarençon D, Masqueliez C, Baubichon D, Galonnier M, Burckhart M-F, Peoc'h M, Mestries JC. Nerve agent poisoning in primates: anti-lethal, anti-epileptic and neuroprotective effects of GK-11. Arch of Toxicol 1998; 72: 84-92.

[27]   Faber NB. Receptor mechanisms and circuitry underlying NMDA antagonist neurotoxicity. Mol Psychi 2002; 7: 32-43.

[28]   Shih TM. Anticonvulsant effects of diazepam and MK-801 in Soman poisoning. Epilepsy Res 1990; 7: 105-116.

[29]   Lallement G,Baubichon D, Didier C, Monique G, Peoc'h M, Carpentier P. Review of the value of gacyclidine (GK-11) as adjuvant medication to conventional treatments of organophosphate poisoning : primate experiments mimicking various scenarios of military or terrorist attack by Soman. NeuroToxicology 1999; 20(4): 675-684.

[30]   Filbert MG, Forster JS, Smith CD, Ballough GP. Neuroprotective effects of HU-211 on brain damage resulting from soman-induced seizures. Ann N Y Acad Sci. 1999; 890: 505-14.

[31]   Sellstrom A. Anticonvulsants in anticholinesterase poisoning. In: Ballantyne B, Marrs TC, Ed. Clinical and experimental toxicology of organophosphates and carbamates. Oxford: Butterworth Heinemann. 1992; pp 578–586.

[32]   Naylor DE, Liu HT, Wasterlain CG. Trafficking of $GABA_A$ receptors, loss of inhibition, and a mechanism for pharmacoresistance in status epilepticus. J Neurosci 2005; 25: 7724 – 7733.

[33]   Rafiq A, DeLorenzo RJ, Coulter DA Generation and propagation of epileptiform discharges in a combined entorhinal cortex/hippocampal slice. J Neurophysiol 1993; 70: 1962–1974.

[34]   MacDonald RL, Kapur J. Acute cellular alterations in the hippocampus after status epilepticus, Epilepsia 1999; 40 (Suppl. I):S9-S20.

[35]   Magnussen I, Oxlund HRW, Alsbirk KE, Arnold E. Absorption of Diazepam in man following rectal and parenteral administration. Acta Pharmacol Toxicol 1979; 45: 87-90.

[36]   Moolenaar F. Bakker S, Visser J, Huizinga T. Biopharmaceutics of rectal administration of drugs in man. IX. Comparative biopharmaceutics of diazepam after single rectal, oral, intramuscular and intravenous administration in Man. Int J Pharm 1980; 5: 127-137.

[37]   Nordgren I, Karlén B, Kimland M, Palmér L, Holmstedt B. Intoxications with anticholinesterases: effect of different combinations of antidotes on the dynamics of acetylcholine in mouse brain. Pharmacol Toxicol 1992; 70: 384-388.

[38]   Ramsay RE, Hammond EJ, Perchalski RJ, Wilder BJ. Brain uptake of phenytoin, phenobarbital and diazepam. Arch Neurol 1979; 36: 535-539.

[39]   Elisabeth R, Tréluyer JM, Pons G. Pharmacokinetic optimisation of benzodiazepine therapy for acute seizures. Clin Pharmacokinet 1999; 36: 409-424.

[40]   Celesia GG, Booker HE, Sato S, Brain and serum concentrations of diazepam in experimental epilepsy. Epilepsia 1974: 15: 417-425.

[41]   Lowenstein DD, Simon RP, Antiepileptic drugs useful in status epilepticus. In : Faingold, C. L.; Fromm, G. H. Ed. Drugs for control of epilepsy: actions on neuronal networks involved in seizure disorders. Boca Raton, FL: CRC Press 1992; pp 513-525.

[42]   Prensky AL, Raff MC, Moore MJ, Schwab RS. Intravenous diazepam in the treatment of prolonged seizure activity. N Engl J Med 1967; 276: 779-784.

[43]   Chiulli DA, Terndrup TE, Kanter RK. The influence of diazepam or lorazepam on the frequency of endotracheal intubation in childhood status epilepticus. J Emerg Med 1991; 9:13–17.

[44]   Shih TM, Tami C. Rowland, McDonough JH, Jr. Anticonvulsants for nerve agent-induced seizures: the influence of the therapeutic dose of atropine. J Pharmacol Exp Ther 2007; 320:154–161.

[45]   McDonough JH Jr, McMonagle J, Copeland T, Zoeffel D, Shih TM. Comparative evaluation of benzodiazepines for control of soman-induced seizures. Arch Toxicol 1999; 73: 473-478.

[46]   Shih TM. Organophosphorus nerve agents, electrographic seizures, anticonvulsants, neuropathology and acute lethality. In : Proceedings of the 2000 U.S. Army Medical Defense Bioscience Review Abstracts 2000, pp 63

[47]   Rotenberg JS, Newmark J. Nerve agent attacks on children: diagnosis and management. Pediatrics 2003;112;648-658

[48]   Chamberlain JM, Altieri MA, Futterman C, Young GM, Ochsenschlager DW, Waisman Y. A prospective, randomized study comparing intramuscular midazolam with intravenous diazepam for treatment of seizures in children. Pediatr Emerg Care 1997; 13: 92-94

[49]   Pellock JM. Use of midazolam for refractory status epilepticus in pediatric patients. J Child Neurol. 1998;13: 581–587.

[50]   Jones DM, Macdonald RL. Characterization of pharmacoresistance to benzodiazepines in the rat Li-pilocarpine model of status epilepticus. Epilepsy Res 2002; 50: 301-312.

[51]   Mazarati AM, Wasterlain CG. Time-dependent decrease in the effectiveness of antiepileptic drugs during the course of self-sustaining status epilepticus. Brain Res 1998; 814: 179-185

[52]   Shih TM, McDonough JH Jr, Koplovitz I. Anticonvulsants for soman-induced seizure activity. J Biomed Sci 1999; 6: 86-96.

[53]   McLeod CG. Pathology of nerve agents: perspectives on medical management. Fundam Appl Toxicol 1985; 5: S10-S16

[54]   Filbert MG, Jaworski J, Hontz B, D. Fath, Walters M, Kan R, Ballough G. A viable neuroprotection strategy following soman-induced status epilepticus. In: Army Medical Research Inst Of Chemical Defense Aberdeen Proving Ground Defense Technical Information Center. ADA443565; 2003.

[55]   Fosbraey P, Wetherell J, French M. Neurotransmitter changes in guinea-pig brain regions following soman intoxication. J Neurochem 1990; 54: 72-79.

[56]   Jacobsson SOP, Cassel GE, Karlsson BM, Sellstrom A, Persson SA. Release of dopamine, GABA and EAA in rats during intrastriatal perfusion with kainic acid, NMDA and Soman: a comparative microdialysis study. Arch Toxicol 1997; 71: 756-765.

[57]   Jacobsson SOP, Cassel GE. Increased levels of nitrogen oxides and lipid peroxidation in the rat brain after soman-induced seizures. Arch Toxicol 1999; 73: 269-273.

[58]   Ennis M, Shipley MT. Tonic activation of locus coeruleus neurons by systemic or intracoerulear microinjection of an irreversible acetylcholinesterase inhibitor: increased discharge rate and induction of c-fos. Exp Neurol 1992; 118: 164-177.

[59]   Etri MME, Nickell WT, Ennis M, Skau KA, Shipley MT. Brain norepinephrine reductions in Soman-intoxicated rats: association with convulsions and ache inhibition, time course, and relation to other monoamines. Exp Neurol 1992; 118: 153-163.

[60]   Rang HP, Dale MM, Ritter JM, Flower R. Chapter 11 - Noradrenergic transmission In: Rang HP, Dale MM, Ritter JM, Flower R. Ed. Rang and Dale's Pharmacology. 6th ed. Churchill Livingstone 2007.

[61]   Libet B, Gleason CA, Wright EW, Feinstein B. Suppression of an epileptiform type of electrocortical activity in the rat by stimulation of the locus coeruleus. Epilepsia 1977; 18: 451-462.

[62]   Curet O. deMontigny C. Electrophysiological characterization of adrenoreceptors in the rat dorsal hippocampus: I. Receptors mediating the effect of microiontophoretically applied norepinephrine. Brain Res 1988; 475:35-46.

[63]   Licata F. Li-Volsi G, Maugeri G, Ciranna L, Santangelo F. Effects of noradrenaline on the firing rate of vestibular neurons. Neuroscience 1993; 475: 35-46.

[64]   Weinshenker D, Szot P. The role of catecholamines in seizure susceptibility: new results using genetically engineered mice. Pharmacol Ther 2002; 94: 213-233.

[65]   Louis WJ, Papanicolaou J, Summers RJ, Vajda FJ. Role of central β-adrenoceptors in the control of pentylenetetrazole-induced convulsions in rats. Br J Pharmacol 1982; 75: 441-446.

[66]   Luchowska E, Luchowski P, Wielosz M, Kleinrok Z, Czuczwar SJ, Urbańska EM. Propranolol and metoprolol enhance the anticonvulsant action of valproate and diazepam against maximal electroshock. Pharmacol Biochem Behav. 2002; 71: 223-231.

[67]   Buccafuso JJ, Aronstam RS. Clonidine protection from the toxicity of soman, an organophosphate acetylcholinesterase inhibitor, in the mouse. J Pharmacol Exp Ther 1986; 239: 43-47.

[68]   Buccafusco JJ, Robert SA. Adrenergic agonists protect against soman, an irreversible acetylcholinesterase inhibitor. Toxicol Lett 1987; 38: 67-76.

[69]   Buccafuso JJ, Graham JH, Aronstam RS. Behavioural effects of toxic doses of soman, protection afforded by clonidine. Pharmacol, Biochem Behav 1988; 29: 309-313.

[70]   Buccafuso JJ, Aronstam RS, Graham JH. Role of central biogenic amines on the protection afforded by clonidine against the toxicity of soman, an irreversible cholinesterase inhibitor. Toxicol Lett 1988; 42: 291-299.

[71]   Magri V, Buccafuso JJ, Aronstam RS. Protection by clonidine from the cardiovascular changes and lethality following soman administration in the rat: role of brain acetylcholine. Toxicol Appl Pharmacol 1988; 95: 464-473.

[72]   Buccafusco JJ. The role of central cholinergic neurons in the regulation of blood pressure and in experimental hypertension. Pharmacol Rev 1996; 48: 179-211

[73]   Szot P, Lester M, Laughlin ML, Palmiter RD, Liles LC, Weinshenker D. The anticonvulsant and proconvulsant effects of α_2-adrenoreceptors agonists are mediated by distinct populations of α_{2a}-adrenoreceptors. Neuroscience 2004; 126: 795-803.

[74]   Collins GGS, McLaughlin NJ. Excitatory and inhibitory effects of noradrenaline on synaptic transmission in rat olfactory cortex slice. Brain Res 1984; 294: 211-223.

[75]   Worek F. Arrhythmias in organophosphate poisoning: effect of atropine and bispyridinium oximes. Arch Int Pharmacodyn Ther 1995; 329: 418-435

[76]   Ballough, GPH, Martin LJ, Cann FJ, Graham JS, Smith CD, Kling CE, Forster JS, Phann S, Filbert MG. Microtubule-associated protein 2 (MAP-2): a sensitive marker of seizure-related brain damage. J Neurosci Methods 1995; 61, 23-32.

[77]   Schmued LC, Albertson C and Slikker W, Jr. Fluoro-Jade: a novel fluorochrome for the sensitive and reliable histochemical localization of neuronal degeneration. Brain Res 1997; 751: 37-46.

[78]   McDonough JH, Jr. Shih TM. Pharmacological modulation of soman-induced seizures. Neurosci Biobehav Rev 1993; 17: 203-215.

[79]   Svensson I, Waara L, Johansson L, Bucht A, Cassel G. Soman-induced interleukin-1β mRNA and protein in rat brain. NeuroToxicology 2001; 22: 355-362.

[80]   Ravizza T, Rizzi M, Perego C, Richichi C, Velísková J, Moshé SL, De Simoni MG, Vezzani A. Inflammatory response and glia activation in developing rat hippocampus after status epilepticus. Epilepsia 2005; 46 (Suppl 5):113-7.

[81]   Zimmer LA, Ennis M, Shipley MT. Soman-induced seizures rapidly activate astrocytes and microglia in discrete brain regions. J Comp Neurol 1997; 378: 482-92.

[82]   Vezzani A, Moneta D, Conti M, Richichi C, Ravizza T, De Luigi A, *et al.* Powerful anticonvulsant action of IL-1 receptor antagonist on intracerebral injection and astrocytic overexpression in mice. Proc Natl Acad Sci USA 2000; 97:11534-9.

CHAPTER 6

Chemically Induced Experimental Models of Absence Epilepsy

Rezzan Gülhan Aker[1,*], Filiz Yilmaz Onat[1,*] and Demet Kinay[2]

[1]*Department of Pharmacology and Clinical Pharmacology, Marmara University School of Medicine, Istanbul, Turkey and* [2]*I. Neurology Clinic, Bakirköy Research Hospital for Neurology, Neurosurgery and Psychiatry, Istanbul, Turkey*

Abstract: Absence epilepsy is a group of syndromes with generalized non-convulsive seizures that are characterized by synchronous spike-and-wave discharges (SWDs) on the electroencephalogram (EEG). Animal models of absence epilepsy generally mimic this non-convulsive type of the absence seizure with SWDs on the EEG. In the literature, there are several experimental *in vitro* and *in vivo* models of the absence epilepsy displaying the spike-and-wave activity induced by different approaches (electrical, chemical, genetic manipulations). All these models have provided valuable insights into the underlying mechanisms and treatment of the disease. The aim of this chapter is to review commonly used *in vivo* animal models of absence seizures that are induced by the administration of chemicals. In these chemical models, SWD activity is induced in an otherwise normal brain.

ABSENCE EPILEPSY

Clinical Considerations

Absence epilepsy is a group of syndromes included among the idiopathic generalized epilepsies and is characterized by non-convulsive seizures which have been classified as typical absence seizures or atypical absence seizures [1].

Absence epilepsy with typical absence seizures is associated with minimal or no long term cognitive impairment [2]. These seizures are manifested clinically by a paroxysmal brief loss of consciousness without aura or postictal state and are associated with generalized, regular 3 Hz spike-and-wave discharges (SWDs) on the electroencephalogram (EEG). Absence epilepsy with typical absence seizures occurs between 4 years of age and adolescence and usually has a benign outcome. It is divided according to the age of onset of the seizures in two forms: childhood absence epilepsy and juvenile absence epilepsy. Juvenile absence epilepsy shows absence seizures with a later onset and longer duration and a greater potential for developing other seizure types compared to childhood absence epilepsy. Typical absence seizures may also occur with other syndromes such as eyelid myoclonia with absences and perioral myoclonia with absences [3].

Absence epilepsy with atypical absence seizures is less common and is generally associated with a severely abnormal cognitive and neurodevelopmental outcome in children [4]. Voluntary behavior during an atypical absence seizure is one of the features that distinguishe atypical from typical absences. Children with atypical absence seizures have an altered state of consciousness but without complete immobility and may be able to walk and talk during the seizure [5]. Atypical absence seizures are more frequent and prolonged than typical absence seizures. The seizure onset and offset of atypical absences are more gradual without the exact concordance between ictal behavior and EEG changes. The frequency of generalized SWDs is slower than 3 Hz in atypical absence seizure.

Pharmacologically, ethosuximide, valproic acid, benzodiazepines (diazepam, clobazam and clonazepam), lamotrigine, topiramate, levetiracetam, zonisamide and GABAB receptor antagonists are effective agents against absence seizures, whereas phenytoin, carbamazepine, oxcarbazepine, vigabatrin, gabapentin, tiagabine or GABAB receptor agonists have no effect or exacerbate absence seizures [6-9].

Drug choice in the treatment of absence epilepsy depends on seizure type and patient age. Ethosuximide, valproic acid, and lamotrigine, alone or in combination, are a first-line therapy in childhood absence epilepsy. Valproic acid

*Address correspondence to Assoc. Prof. Rezzan Gülhan Aker and Prof. Filiz Yilmaz Onat:** Department of Pharmacology and Clinical Pharmacology, Marmara University School of Medicine, Istanbul, Turkey; Tel: 009-02163492816; E-mails: raker@marmara.edu.tr, fonat@marmara.edu.tr

is preferred for juvenile absence epilepsy because it reduces the high probability of developing lifelong myoclonic jerks and generalized tonic-clonic seizures, which is greater than for childhood absence epilepsy [6]. When there is concern about teratogenicity, lamotrigine can be given as a first-line monotherapy, although onset of action is much slower compared to valproic acid. Valproic acid controls absences in 75% of patients and has the advantage also of controlling generalized tonic-clonic seizures (70%) and myoclonic jerks (75%); however it may be undesirable for women considering pregnancy. Ethosuximide controls 70% of absences, but does not protect children against tonic-clonic seizures, so that it is unsuitable as monotherapy when other generalized seizures coexist Lamotrigine may control absences and generalized tonic-clonic seizures in possibly 50% to 60% of patients, although it may worsen myoclonic jerks; skin rashes are common [6].

A recent clinical study comparing the efficacy, tolerability, and neuropsychological effects of ethosuximide, valproic acid and lamotrigine in children with newly diagnosed childhood absence epilepsy showed that ethosuximide and valproic acid were more effective than lamotrigine in suppressing absence seizures and ethosuximide was associated with fewer adverse attentional effects as compared with valproic acid [10]. A combination of any of these three drugs may be needed for resistant cases [6].

Mechanism

Both human and animal studies indicated that hypersynchronisation within thalamocortical circuits generates SWDs in absence seizures [11]. However, there are reports indicating that brain regions beyond the thalamocortical networks participate in some aspects of typical absence seizures, such as metabolic changes, or increases in synchronization between hippocampi during SWDs [12-14]. In contrast to this, atypical absence seizures involve both thalamocortical and limbic circuitry according to some evidence from experimental, clinical and neuroimaging studies [14, 15].

Main components of the thalamocortical circuit generating SWDs in typical absence seizures include the reticular and ventrobasal (ventroposteromedial, ventroposterolateral) nuclei of the thalamus and somatosensory cortex (especially the perioral region) [2, 7, 16-17]. In this circuitry, hyperexcitability of the cortex and increase in GABAergic tonus and in the amplitude of T-type calcium currents activated by hyperpolarization in the thalamus are important key features. Basically, there are reciprocal excitatory glutamatergic projections between cortex and thalamus. These neurons send axon collaterals to the reticular nucleus of the thalamus, which consists mainly of GABA containing neurons projecting both to each other and to the thalamic relay nuclei. These neurons can produce both tonic and burst firing and can generate rhythmic oscillations such as sleep spindles. Activation of the reticular nucleus of the thalamus can lead to a burst of synchronized firing of GABAergic neurons, causing inhibitory postsynaptic potentials (IPSPs) in thalamocortical neurons. GABA induced hyperpolarization, especially through $GABA_B$ receptors in the specific relay nuclei and the reticular nuclei of the thalamus, results in low-voltage activated T-type calcium currents that create a rebound burst of fast spikes leading to the next cycle of the oscillation. Recent evidence from genetic models in rats of absence epilepsy suggests that a specific group of neurons in somatosensory cortex starts firing during the first 500 ms of the SWDs and drives related thalamic nuclei and cortex on to the oscillation [18]. After the first milliseconds, both cortex and thalamus drive each other resulting in the amplification and maintenance of rhythmic SWDs. Another study reported that the neurons of the focus area are in cortical layers 5/6 of the perioral region [19]. Several alterations in this circuitry have been described at the level of receptors ($GABA_A$ and $GABA_B$ receptors in the thalamus) and ion channels (voltage-gated Na+ channels in the cortex, low-voltage activated T-type calcium channels, hyperpolarization-activated cyclic-nucleotide-gated cation channels (HCN)) in various models [20].

Animal Models

Animal models of absence epilepsy, like any models of a disease should be reproducible, predictable, and quantifiable. They have to show comparable electrophysiology, behavior, etiology, pathophysiology as well as a pharmacological response profile that is comparable to human absence epilepsy. There are several in-vivo models of absence epilepsy that are induced by electrical stimulation, chemical injections or genetic manipulations in different species from drosophila to non-human primates including baboons, cats, rats and mice [21-24]. However not every model fulfills all these criteria (Table 1). The main common feature of these absence epilepsy models is the hypersynchronization in thalamo-cortical circuitry that results in the production of bilaterally synchronous bursts that are similar to the spike-and-wave activity on the EEG that is seen in the human form. However, the frequency of the spike-and-wave activity in animal models differs depending on the mode of seizure induction and the species. Therefore one should select the model depending on its limitations and on the nature of the question under consideration.

This chapter will focus on the most commonly used *in vivo* models of absence epilepsy induced by chemical administrations. The majority of them are in fact absence seizure (ictogenesis) models having bilateral synchronous bursts similar to spike-and-wave activity on the EEG.

Table 1: Characteristics of Typical Human Childhood Absence Epilepsy and of the Animal Model Correlates Induced by Chemicals.

Criteria	Typical childhood absence epilepsy	Chemical model
Etiology	Idiopathic (genetic)	-
Mechanism	Thalamo-cortical circuit	FGPE, L-PTZ, GHB
Age of onset	Childhood	-
Remission	Adolescence	-
Electrophysiological pattern	Bilaterally synchronous SWD	FGPE, L-PTZ, GHB, THIP
Behavioral characteristic	Behavioral arrest, loss of consciousness,	FGPE, L-PTZ, GHB
Pharmacologic response	Suppressed by ethosuximide and valproic acid	FGPE, L-PTZ, GHB

SWD: spike-and-wave discharge, FGPE: feline generalized penicillin epilepsy, L-PTZ: low dose pentylenetetrazole, GHB: gamma-hydroxy butyrate, THIP: tetrahydroxyisoxazolo pyridine

CHEMICALLY INDUCED EXPERIMENTAL MODELS OF ABSENCE EPILEPSY

Chemical models are usually defined as acute models rather than chronic, therefore they should be regarded as seizure or ictogenesis models. They are induced by acute administration, locally into the cerebrum or systemically by subcutaneous, intramuscular, intraperitoneal or intravenous injections, of a specific substance that has a limited duration of action [25-26]. The seizures are observed within a specific time frame. Bilaterally synchronous cortical activity resembling SWDs generally correlates with the behavior of the animal (mostly behavioral arrest, sometimes twitching of vibrissae and facial myoclonus). Seizures start and end abruptly in the EEG with a normal background activity. The duration and the frequency of the SWDs vary in relation to species and chemical substance.

There are several chemical substances used locally (into the brain) or systemically to induce absence seizures. The most commonly studied models of typical absence epilepsy include the feline generalized penicillin epilepsy model (FGPE), the low-dose pentylenetetrazole (L-PTZ) model, the 4,5,6,7 tetrahydroxyisoxazolo (4,5,c) pyridine 3-ol (THIP) model, and the gamma-hydroxy butyrate (GHB) model. There are two models for atypical absence epilepsy. These are the AY-9944 and the methylazoxymethanol acetate (MAM)-AY-9944 models. There are also a few reports of different models of epilepsy associated with absence seizures such as the muscimol-induced absence seizure model [27], the intraventricular opiate model [28] and unilateral kainic acid injection into the mediodorsal nucleus of the thalamus [29], which are not included in this chapter. We refer interested readers to these specific publications since these models are also quite interesting with special features that should be considered.

Models of Typical Absence Epilepsy

1. Systemic Penicillin: The Feline Generalized Penicillin Epilepsy Model (FGPE).

Antibiotics, for instance the penicillins (benzyl penicillin, phenoxymethylpenicillin, oxacillin, methicillin, ampicillin) and cephalosporins can produce seizures when applied locally onto cortex or administered systemically at high doses. Penicillins (see Table **2**, panel 8 for chemical structure) owe their convulsant activity through selective antagonism of GABA-mediated postsynaptic inhibition [30].

In cats, intramuscular administration of a high dose of penicillin (250.000-600.000 Units/kg) produces seizures with SWDs that fulfill the criteria for the experimental models of generalized absence epilepsy (Table **1**) [23, 31]. Seizures start about 1 hour after the injection and last 4-8 hours. Intravenously, lower doses (50.000-100.000 IU/kg) evoke similar activity within 30 minutes with a much higher propensity for generalized tonic-clonic seizures. Behavioral arrest, blinking, myoclonus of face and neck muscles are observed in freely moving animals. The SWD frequency in the FGPE model is 3-5 Hz, similar to that of the human form of typical absence seizures. However in rodents, intramuscular penicillin administration produces multifocal spikes and occasionally bilaterally synchronous spike-and-wave activity [31].

Formerly, FGPE was one of the most studied models of absence epilepsy. It was first described by Prince and Farell during the 1969 meeting of American Academy of Neurology [32]. Thereafter it was widely studied. The mechanisms that generate generalized absence seizures through both cortical and thalamic interactions, the pharmacologic characteristics and their differences from focal seizures were described. Studies of this model suggested that SWDs evolved from sleep spindles and that both cortex and thalamus were essential for producing generalized SWDs (Fig. **1**). In the underlying mechanism proposed cortical pyramidal neurons, under the influence of excitatory post-synaptic potentials (EPSPs) conveyed by thalamocortical volleys, recruit intracortical recurrent inhibitory interneurons and this results in sleep spindles. In the FGPE

Table 2: The chemical structures of the agents used to model absence epilepsy.

1. GABA	2. GHB
3. GBL	4. THIP (Gaboxadol)
5. Bicucculline	6. Picrotoxin
	picrotoxinin picrotin
7. PTZ	8. Penicillin G

1. AY-9944

The chemical structure of gama-amino butyric acid (GABA); of GABA$_A$ receptor agonists GHB, GBL, THIP (panels 2, 3 and 4); of GABA$_A$ receptor antagonists bicucculline, PTZ, picrotoxin (panels 5, 6, and 7), Penicillin G (panel 8) and of AY-9944, a cholesterol synthesis inhibitor (panel 9). Abbreviations: GHB: gamma-hydroxy butyrate; GBL: gamma butyrolactone; PTZ: pentylenetetrazole; THIP: 4,5,6,7 tetrahydroxyisoxazolo (4,5,c) pyridine 3-ol.

model, due to the penicillin-induced hyperexcitability of the cortex, summation of the EPSPs of thalamocortical volleys in the cortical neurons results in the transformation of spindle-waves into spikes of SWDs and the slow-wave component develops as a result of the summation of intracortical IPSPs. It was also suggested that the cortex initiated the SWDs and thalamus followed the cortex in a phase–locked manner to produce the oscillatory pattern. However, inactivation of either cortex or thalamus abolished the generalized SWDs suggesting that both together were essential to produce generalized SWDs. All of these findings provided an experimental basis for the "Corticoreticular Theory" conceptualized by Gloor and opened an era that provided further research on the mechanisms of SWDs. Today although this hypothesis has been challenged with new findings on the origin of SWDs in several other models, it still plays an important role in inspiring further research on the topic (31, 33).

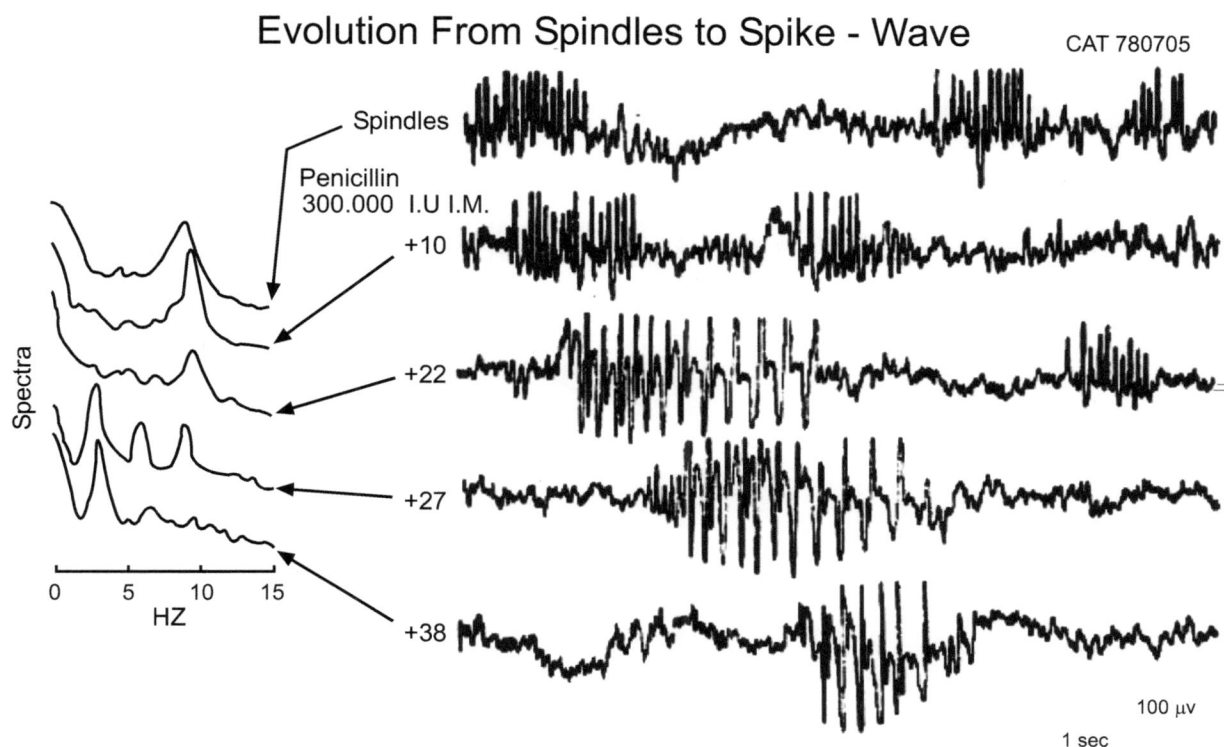

Figure 1: Representative cortical EEG recording showing a gradual development of SWDs from sleep spindles in the FGPE model (Reproduced with permission from Kostopoulos, 2000 [33]).

Low Dose Pentylenetetrazole (L-PTZ) Model

Pentylentetrazole (PTZ) acts mainly through central GABAA receptors. It binds to the t-butyl-bicyclo-phosphorothionate (TBPS) site of the receptor and blocks GABAergic neurotransmission [34] thus decreasing the inhibitory effects of GABA. It can produce seizures in several species including frogs, mice, rats, monkeys and humans in a dose-dependent manner [26]. Low doses (10-30 mg/kg given intraperitoneally or subcutaneously) produce 'freezing' and myoclonic jerks, twitching of vibrissae with rhythmic 6-7 Hz spike-and-wave activity on the EEG in mice and rats (see video-1 in supplementary files). Clonic and tonic-clonic seizures develop with higher doses (50-100 mg/kg). Seizures start shortly after the injection within 2-10 minutes depending on the dose and species (Table **3**). The mean duration of each SWD complex is 2-3 sec in Wistar rats treated with 20 mg/kg PTZ (i.p.), the number of seizures reaches a maximum within 60 minutes and wanes within 4 hours (Fig. **2**).

Everett and Richards, in 1944, demonstrated that trimetadione and phenobarbital but not phenytoin blocked seizures induced by PTZ. Since then, PTZ has been used for the screening of anti-epileptic drugs along with the maximal electroshock seizure (MES) test [35]. The suppression of seizures or an increase in latency to the induction of behavioral and electroencephalographic features produced by a PTZ injection is regarded as signifying a possible anti-absence activity of the substance being tested.

GABA$_A$ receptor antagonists such as bicuculline and picrotoxin produce seizures which are similar to PTZ seizures. The chemical structures of these GABA$_A$ receptor antagonists are presented in table 2 (panels 5, 6 and 7). All these substances induce behavioral arrest, clonus and tonic-clonic seizures within a continuum in a dose dependent manner. PTZ is preferred to the others because it is easier to use and is more reliable than bicuculline or picrotoxin (for example, for titration of the dose, dissolving the drug, and latency to seizure induction).

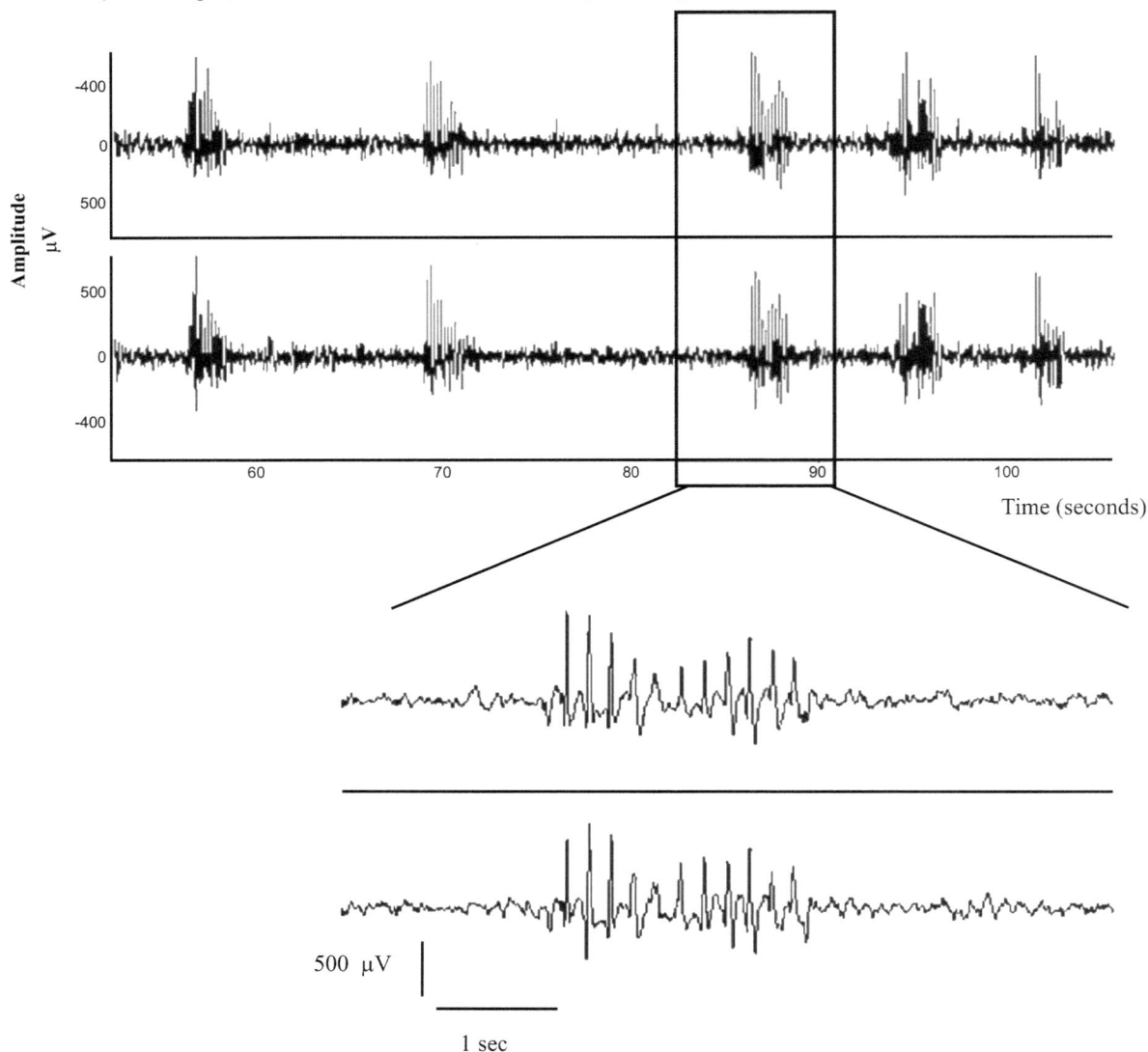

Figure 2: Representative cortical EEG trace recorded from an adult Wistar rat administrered PTZ (20 mg/kg, i.p). Top traces show bilaterally synchronous bursts recorded from left and right cortices. Below is the enlargement of the selected part.

Gamma-Hydroxy-Butyrate (GHB) and Gamma-Butyrolactone (GBL) Model

Experimental chemical models of absence epilepsy defined by EEG, behavioral and pharmacological characteristics include the administration of gamma-hydroxybutyrate (GHB) or gamma-butyrolactone (GBL) (their chemical structures are shown in Table **2** -panels 2 and 3). The GHB and GBL models meet the criteria of having EEG, behavioral and pharmacological profiles similar to those of human absence epilepsy (Table **3**) [2]. Absence seizures are produced by acute or chronic repeated administration of GHB or GBL usually to a rat or mouse which are the most readily available laboratory animals for these models. GHB is a sedative-hypnotic agent and was earlier used clinically in the treatment of narcolepsy and alcoholism as well as an adjuvant agent in general anesthesia [36]. Later on GHB became popular as a recreational drug with addictive properties and therefore is a legally controlled substance [37].

Figure 3: GBL induced seizure activity in a Wistar rat. The inset figures show the power spectrum of selected seizure activities with a peak frequency of 4.8 Hz in the first injection and 5.8 Hz in the 18th injection.

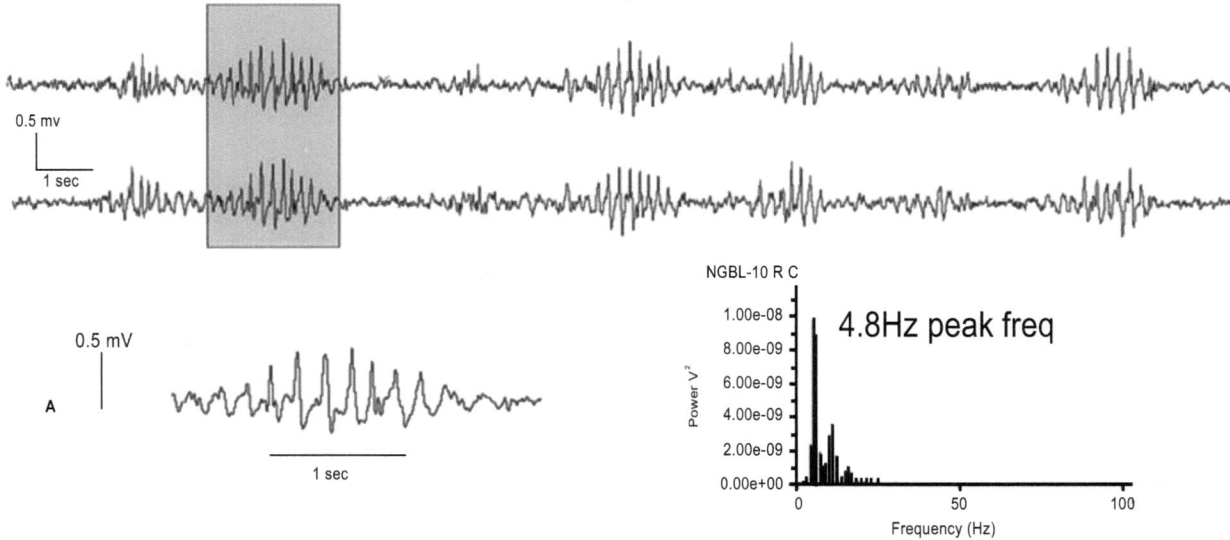

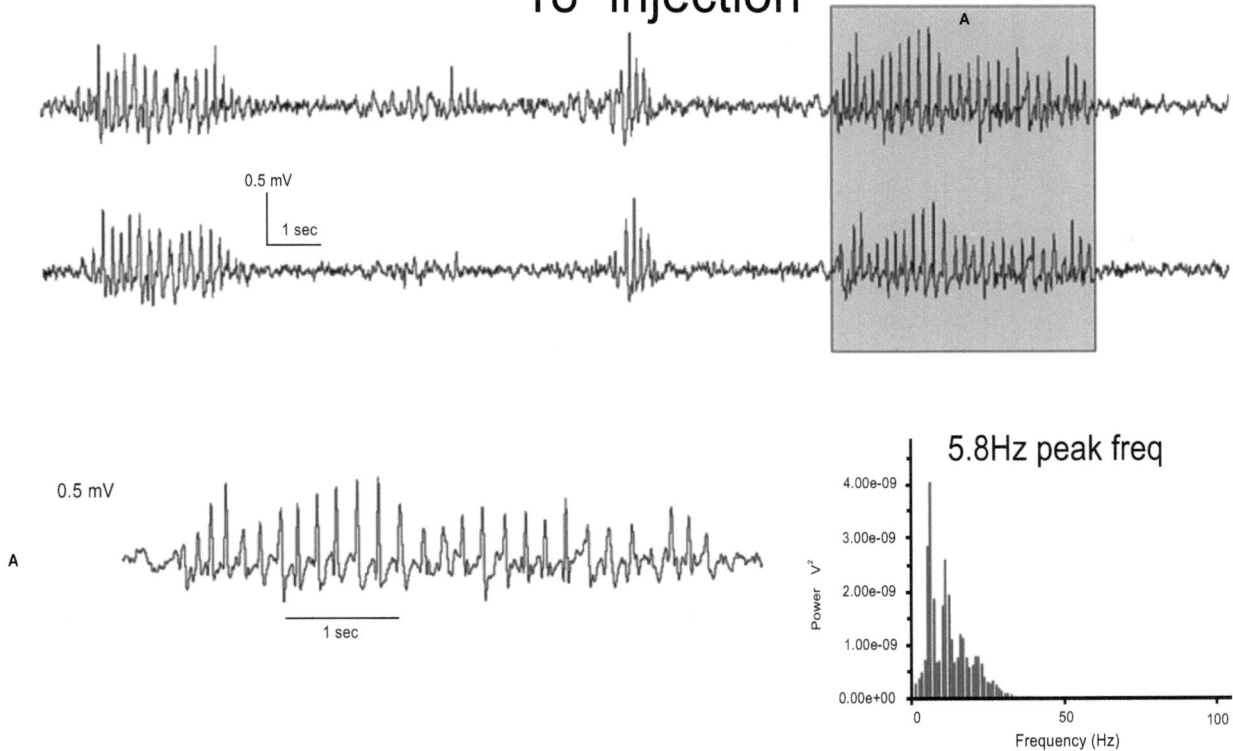

GHB has been known as a naturally occurring endogenous substance in the mammalian central nervous system since the 1960s [38]. Endogenous GHB is present in small concentrations in many brain regions and in extra-neuronal peripheral tissues [39]. The primary precursor of endogenous GHB in the brain is GABA which is converted either by an oxidative pathway as a main route or by a reductive pathway through succinic semialdehyde [40]. Studies of the regional distribution of GHB binding sites by autoradiographic techniques have shown the presence of GHB receptors in the cortex, striatum, hippocampus, thalamus, hypothalamus and substantia nigra [40, 41]. A number of studies have reported the affinity of GHB for $GABA_B$ receptors and have demonstrated that GHB acts on thalamo-cortical neurons through the activation of $GABA_B$ receptors [42-44]. However, recent molecular evidence shows the existence of a GHB receptor that is distinct from the GABAB receptors [45]. NCS-382 has been used as a GHB receptor antagonist [46], but it also has a number of non-specific actions on synaptic currents [43].

GHB and GBL, when administered parenterally, easily cross the blood brain barrier and enter the mammalian brain. GBL used as a GHB precursor is readily and irreversibly transformed by peripheral tissue to GHB. GBL has the advantage of a more rapid onset of action and a predictable dose responserelationship compared to GHB [47]. Both GHB and GBL can be administered systemically in a dose range of 50-400 mg/kg by different routes including intravenously, intraperitoneally, and subcutaneously to a number of species [2, 48]. A systemic injection of GHB (62.5-375 mg/kg) or GBL (85-170 mg/kg) to Genetic Absence Epilepsy Rats From Strasbourg (GAERS) produces a dose-dependent increase in the cumulative SWD durations (48). Exogenous applications of GHB and GBL lead to absence seizures through potentiation of the GHB-related neuromodulation and/or interaction with GABAergic inhibitory and excitatory neurotransmissions in cortico-thalamo-cortical circuit. Electrophysiological *in vitro* slice studies have shown that SWDs are evoked within a narrow range of GHB concentrations (240–500 μM) applied to the ventrobasal thalamocortical neurons of a rat; higher concentrations produce a progressive slowing of the EEG associated with increasingly strong sedation and sleep [43, 49].

Intraperitoneal administration of 100 mg/kg of GBL to an adult Wistar rat produces a rapid onset of bilaterally synchronous paroxysms in the cortical EEG accompanied by immobility, vacant-staring and sometimes vibrissal twitching (see video-1 in supplementary files). These paroxysms at 4-6 cycles per second consist of bursts of spikes together with spike-and-wave components after the first injections. These GBL-induced discharges were similar to the paroxysms observed in 30 day postnatal old GAERS [50]. They start to appear 4.8±0.5 min after the injection, reach maximum numbers and durations within 20 minutes and return to the baseline EEG 90 min after the injection (Fig. **3**). Repeated injections, twice a day over 10 days, result in a higher frequency (5-7 cycles per second) and higher amplitude discharges relative to the ones observed after the first administrations (Fig. **3**). Additionally residual spike and spike-and-wave paroxysms can be observed 48-72 hours after repeated injections [unpublished observation by Onat].

An analysis of the mouse thalamic proteome using fluorescence 2D difference gel electrophoresis combined with mass spectrometry showed reversible changes in the expression of particular proteins corresponding to the appearance of SWDs 10 min after the intraperitoneal administration of 50 mg/kg GBL and these returned back to their original levels 30 min after the injection [51]. Similarly, an alteration of GluR2 protein expression in the cerebral cortex has been reported following 100 mg/kg GBL-induced absence seizures in rats [52].

Tetrahydroxyisoxazolo Pyridine (THIP) Model

4,5,6,7 tetrahydroxyisoxazolo (4,5,c) pyridine 3-ol (THIP, chemical structure is illustrated in Table **2**-panel 4) is a selective agonist for the extrasynaptic GABAA receptors containing delta-subunits which are insensitive to benzodiazepines. These receptors were found abundantly in thalamus, hippocampus and neocortex [53].

Experimentally, THIP can be administered intraperitoneally at a dose of 5-10 mg/kg in rats. Spike-and-wave like activity occurs in bursts that last 1-9 seconds. This model is used for its electroclinical features that correlate with absence seizures rather than the pharmacological characteristics. THIP increases SWDs when administered to GAERS, and though controversially, valproic acid potentiates the aggravating effects of THIP on SWDs [54].

THIP was in clinical development by the drug companies Lundbeck and Merck for the treatment of insomnia and was named gaboxadol. Clinically, gaboxadol was shown to increase total sleep time, improve sleep maintenance and the slow wave sleep phase in patients with primary insomnia without a clear effect on sleep onset. However, the clinical development was discontinued in phase III because of limited or variable efficacy and the occurrence of psychiatric side effects at supratherapeutic doses in an abuse liability study that involved drug abusers [55].

Table 3: Characteristics Of Typical Human Childhood Absence Epilepsy And The Animal Model Correlates Induced By Chemicals.

Features		Typical Absence Seizures					Atypical Absence Seizures	
		Animal Model				Human	Animal Model	Human
		FGPE	L-PTZ	GHB	THIP	CTAE	AY-9944	CAAS
General	Species (frequently used)	Cat	Rat, mice	Rat	Rat	Human	Rat	Human
	Strain	ND	SD,W	SD,W, LE	W	NA	LE	NA
	Procedure	IM	IP, SC	IP	IP	NA	SC	NA
	Dose (mg/kg)	300.000-600.000 U	10-30	100 (GBL)	10	NA	7,5	NA
	Latency (min)	30-60	2—20	3—5	4—5	Spontaneous	Spontaneous	Spontaneous
	Reproducibility	YES	YES	YES	YES	NA	YES	NA
	Standardized, quantitative	YES	YES	YES	YES	NA	YES	NA
	Other Seizure Types	YES	NO	NO	NO	NO	YES	YES
	Cognitive deficits	NO	NO	NO	ND	NO	YES	YES
SWD	Bilaterally synchronous	YES	YES	YES	YES	YES	YES	YES
	Frequency (Hz)	3-5	7—9	4-8	7—9	2,5-4	4—6	1,5-3
	Recordings from thalamus and cortex	YES	YES	YES	ND	YES	YES	ND
	Recordings from hippocampus	NO	NO	NO	ND	ND	YES	ND
Behavior	Immobility, staring and myoclonus	YES	YES	YES	YES	YES	YES	YES
	EEG/behavioral correlation	YES	YES	YES	YES	YES	NO	NO
	Movement during SWD	NO	NO	NO	NO	NO	YES	YES
Pharmacology	Blocked by ETX, VPA, TMD	YES	YES	YES	YES	YES	YES	YES
	Exacerbated by GABA$_{A,B}$ receptor agonists	YES	YES	YES	YES	YES	YES	YES

SWD: spike-and-wave discharge, FGPE: feline generalized penicillin epilepsy, L-PTZ: low dose pentylenetetrazole, GHB: gama-hydroxy butyrate, THIP: tetrahydroxyisoxazolo pyridine, ETX: ethosuximide, VPA: valproic acid, TMD: trimetadion, SD: Sprague-Dawley, W: Wistar, LE: Long Evans, ND: not defined, NA: not applicable.

Models of Atypical Absence Epilepsy

1. AY-9944 model. Atypical absence seizures, are less common than the typical ones and have abnormal cognitive and neurodevelopmental outcomes in humans. They can be mimicked by the cholesterol synthesis inhibitor, AY-9944. After early postnatal inhibition of cholesterol synthesis with repeated AY-9944 administration, rats present behavioral and cognitive manifestations similar to the symptoms associated with atypical seizures in children [15, 56]. One protocol for producing this model in rats includes treatment with subcutaneous injections of 7.5 mg/kg of AY-9944 every 6 days from postnatal day 2 to postnatal day 33 [15]. It was also shown that a single injection of AY-9944 at postnatal day 5 or 11 can lead to an atypical absence seizure-like phenotype) [57-58]. Spontaneous, recurrent seizures are observed starting by postnatal day 21 and persist throughout the life of the animal with a peak in adulthood. SWDs are not time-locked with the ictal behavior and the frequency is lower than in the other rat models of absence seizures resembling the human condition of atypical absence seizures. Pharmacologically SWDs are diminished or disappear with ethosuximide and valproat treatments and are exacerbated by phenytoin and GABA agonists [15]. Besides the cortico-thalamo-cortical circuitry, the involvement of hippocampal circuitry has also been shown in this model [14]. Another interesting finding was that the early postnatal treatment with AY-9944 disturbed incorporation of GABAA and GABAB receptor proteins into the lipid rafts of the membrane without disturbing the lipid rafts. This shift may have an effect on the functional development of GABA receptors at their very critical "switch" period between excitatory and inhibitory neurotransmission that may contribute epileptogenesis in this chronic atypical absence epilepsy model [58].

These findings indicating new mechanisms for epileptogenesis and new therapeutic targets for drug development may lead to new strategies in the diagnosis and treatment of epilepsy.

Methylazoxymethanol Acetate (MAM)-AY Model

Recently, a model for atypical absence seizures intractable to treatment with classical antiabsence drugs was described. Administration of AY-9944 (as described above) during postnatal development in rats which were exposed prenatally to MAM (25 mg/kg, ip, at gestational day 15) resulted in a chronic model with spontaneous, recurrent, bilaterally synchronous slow SWD seizures which were refractory to ethosuximide, sodium valproate, and the GABAB receptor antagonist CGP 35348, and were exacerbated by carbamazepine [59].

MAM is an antimitotic agent acting through methylation of pyrimidine bases within 2-24 hours of administration. It is used to model neuronal migration disorders in rats. Its effect on selected neuronal populations depends on the time of administration during gestation. When administered prenatally on gestational day 15, it results in ataxia, tremors, learning and memory impairment, susceptibility to seizures induced by chemicals, dysgenesis, heteretopias and abnormal neuronal activity in the hippocampus and neocortex although no spontaneous seizures are observed in the rat pups [60]. However, combination of MAM with AY-9944 generated a promising model for refractory atypical absence seizures which usually have poor neurodevelopment prognosis. This model can also be a tool for the development of new antiepileptic drugs for the patients who do not respond to current medications available for the treatment of epilepsy.

FUTURE RESEARCH DIRECTIONS

Chemical models, as described above, imitate electro-clinical, behavioral and/or pharmacological features of absence epilepsy. They have provided valuable information on how epileptic discharges, particularly generalized SWDs, occur in otherwise normal brain and on the structures involved in these generalized activities. They have also served in the search and the development of new antiepileptic drugs as well as in an understanding of their mechanism of action. However these models have some limitations as well. For example, the seizures are not spontaneous, except in models of atypical absence epilepsy, and are closely related to the pharmacologic activity of the applied agent. Considering that epilepsy is a multifactorial chronic disorder, there is a need for new methods that would allow studies of this complex interaction of underlying mechanisms and epileptogenesis, which would lead to new and better tools for diagnosis, seizure prediction, surrogate markers and effective therapies. Chemical models such as of atypical absence seizures are close to these criteria and can be used much more efficiently in future research to get answers for the above issues that are also stressed in the International League against Epilepsy (ILAE)-2008 research priorities position paper "Research Priorities in Epilepsy for the Next Decade"[61].

ACKNOWLEDGEMENT

The authors thank R.W. Guillery for his valuable comments on the manuscript.

REFERENCES

[1]   Berg AT, Berkovic SF, Brodie MJ *et al.* Revised terminology and concepts for organization of seizures and epilepsies: report of the ILAE Commission on Classification and Terminology, 2005-2009. Epilepsia 2010; 51: 676-85.

[2]   Snead OC, 3rd. Basic mechanisms of generalized absence seizures. Ann Neurol 1995; 37: 146-57.

[3]   Panayiotopoulos CP, Obeid T, Waheed G. Differentiation of typical absence seizures in epileptic syndromes. A video EEG study of 224 seizures in 20 patients. Brain 1989;112 (Pt 4): 1039-56.

[4]   Markand ON. Lennox-Gastaut syndrome (childhood epileptic encephalopathy). J Clin Neurophysiol 2003; 20: 426-41.

[5]   Nolan M, Bergazar M, Chu B, Cortez MA, Snead OC, 3rd. Clinical and neurophysiologic spectrum associated with atypical absence seizures in children with intractable epilepsy. J Child Neurol 2005; 20: 404-10.

[6]   Panayiotopoulos CP. Treatment of typical absence seizures and related epileptic syndromes. Paediatr Drugs 2001; 3: 379-403.

[7]   Manning JP, Richards DA, Bowery NG. Pharmacology of absence epilepsy. Trends Pharmacol Sci 2003; 24: 542-9.

[8]   Goren MZ, Onat F. Ethosuximide: from bench to bedside. CNS Drug Rev 2007; 13: 224-39.

[9]   Raspall-Chaure M, Neville BG, Scott RC. The medical management of the epilepsies in children: conceptual and practical considerations. Lancet Neurol 2008; 7: 57-69.

[10]   Glauser TA, Cnaan A, Shinnar S, Hirtz DG, Dlugos D, Masur D, *et al.* Ethosuximide, valproic acid, and lamotrigine in childhood absence epilepsy. N Engl J Med 2010; 362: 790-9.

[11]   Snead OC, 3rd, Depaulis A, Vergnes M, Marescaux C. Absence epilepsy: advances in experimental animal models. Adv Neurol 1999; 79: 253-78.

[12]   Nehlig A, Vergnes M, Boyet S, Marescaux C. Metabolic activity is increased in discrete brain regions before the occurrence of spike-and-wave discharges in weanling rats with genetic absence epilepsy. Brain Res Dev Brain Res 1998; 108: 69-75.

[13]   Nehlig A, Vergnes M, Boyet S, Marescaux C. Local cerebral glucose utilization in adult and immature GAERS. Epilepsy Res 1998; 32: 206-12.

[14]   Velazquez JL, Huo JZ, Dominguez LG, Leshchenko Y, Snead OC, 3rd. Typical versus atypical absence seizures: network mechanisms of the spread of paroxysms. Epilepsia 2007; 48: 1585-93.

[15]   Cortez MA, McKerlie C, Snead OC, 3rd. A model of atypical absence seizures: EEG, pharmacology, and developmental characterization. Neurology 2001; 56: 341-9.

[16]   Marescaux C, Vergnes M, Depaulis A. Genetic absence epilepsy in rats from Strasbourg--a review. J Neural Transm Suppl 1992; 35: 37-69.

[17]   Meeren H, van Luijtelaar G, Lopes da Silva F, Coenen A. Evolving concepts on the pathophysiology of absence seizures: the cortical focus theory. Arch Neurol 2005; 62: 371-6.

[18]   Meeren HK, Pijn JP, Van Luijtelaar EL, Coenen AM, Lopes da Silva FH. Cortical focus drives widespread corticothalamic networks during spontaneous absence seizures in rats. J Neurosci 2002; 22: 1480-95.

[19]   Polack PO, Guillemain I, Hu E, Deransart C, Depaulis A, Charpier S. Deep layer somatosensory cortical neurons initiate spike-and-wave discharges in a genetic model of absence seizures. J Neurosci 2007; 27: 6590-9.

[20]   Budde T, Pape HC, Kumar SS, Huguenard JR. Thalamic, thalamocortical, and corticocortical models of epilepsy with an emphasis on absence seizures. In: Pitkanen A, Moshe S, Schwartzkroin P, Eds. Models of Seizures and Epilepsy. Academic Press 2006; pp. 73-88.

[21]   Fisher RS. Animal models of the epilepsies. Brain Res Brain Res Rev. 1989;14: 245-78.

[22]   Engel J. Experimental animal models of epilepsy: classification and relevance to human epileptic phenomena. Epilepsy Res Suppl 1992; 8: 9-20.

[23]   Sarkisian MR. Overview of the Current Animal Models for Human Seizure and Epileptic Disorders. Epilepsy Behav 2001; 2: 201-16.

[24]   Pitkanen A, Moshe, S., Schwartkroin, P., Eds. Models of Seizures and Epilepsy. Academic Press; 2006.

[25]   Marcus EM. Experimental Models of Petit Mal Epilepsy. In: Purpura DP, Penry, J.K., Tower, D., Woodbury, D.M., Walter, R., Eds. Experimetal Models of Epilepsy- A Manual for the Laboratory Worker. New York: Raven Press 1972; pp. 113-46.

[26]   Velisek L. Models of Chemically-Induced Acute Seizures. In: Pitkanen A, Moshe, S., Schwartkroin, P., editor. Models of Seizures and Epilepsy. Academic Press 2006; pp. 127-52.

[27]   Zhang X, Le Gal La Salle G, Ridoux V, Yu PH, Ju G. Fos oncoprotein expression in the rat forebrain following muscimol-induced absence seizures. Neurosci Lett 1996; 210: 169-72.

[28]   Snead OC, 3rd, Bearden LJ. The epileptogenic spectrum of opiate agonists. Neuropharmacology 1982; 21: 1137-44.

[29]   Kato K, Urino T, Hori T *et al.* Experimental petit mal-like seizure induced by microinjection of kainic acid into the unilateral mediodorsal nucleus of the thalamus. Neurol Med Chir (Tokyo) 2008 ; 48: 285-90.

[30]   Macdonald RL, Barker JL. Specific antagonism of GABA-mediated postsynaptic inhibition in cultured mammalian spinal cord neurons: a common mode of convulsant action. Neurology 1978; 28: 325-30.

[31]   Avoli M. Feline generalized penicillin epilepsy. Ital J Neurol Sci 1995; 16: 79-82.

[32]   Prince DA, Farrell, D. Centrencephalic spikewave discharges following parenteral penicillin injection in the cat. Neurology 1969; 19: 309-10.

[33]   Kostopoulos GK. Spike-and-wave discharges of absence seizures as a transformation of sleep spindles: the continuing development of a hypothesis. Clin Neurophysiol 2000; 111(Suppl 2): S27-38.

[34]   Olsen RW. The GABA postsynaptic membrane receptor-ionophore complex. Site of action of convulsant and anticonvulsant drugs. Mol Cell Biochem 1981; 39: 261-79.

[35]   White HS, Johnson M, Wolf HH, Kupferberg HJ. The early identification of anticonvulsant activity: role of the maximal electroshock and subcutaneous pentylenetetrazol seizure models. Ital J Neurol Sci 1995; 16: 73-7.

[36]   Wong CG, Gibson KM, Snead OC, 3rd. From the street to the brain: neurobiology of the recreational drug gamma-hydroxybutyric acid. Trends Pharmacol Sci 2004; 25: 29-34.

[37]   Bernasconi R, Mathivet P, Bischoff S, Marescaux C. Gamma-hydroxybutyric acid: an endogenous neuromodulator with abuse potential? Trends Pharmacol Sci 1999; 20: 135-41.

[38]   Bessman SP, Fishbein WN. Gamma-Hydroxybutyrate, a Normal Brain Metabolite. Nature 1963; 200: 1207-8.

[39]   Nelson T, Kaufman E, Kline J, Sokoloff L. The extraneural distribution of gamma-hydroxybutyrate. J Neurochem. 1981; 37: 1345-8.

[40]   Maitre M. The gamma-hydroxybutyrate signalling system in brain: organization and functional implications. Prog Neurobiol 1997; 51: 337-61.

[41]   Benavides J, Rumigny JF, Bourguignon JJ *et al.* High affinity binding sites for gamma-hydroxybutyric acid in rat brain. Life Sci 1982; 30: 953-61.

[42]   Erhardt S, Andersson B, Nissbrandt H, Engberg G. Inhibition of firing rate and changes in the firing pattern of nigral dopamine neurons by gamma-hydroxybutyric acid (GHBA) are specifically induced by activation of GABA(B) receptors. Naunyn Schmiedebergs Arch Pharmacol 1998; 357: 611-9.

[43]   Gervasi N, Monnier Z, Vincent P *et al.* Pathway-specific action of gamma-hydroxybutyric acid in sensory thalamus and its relevance to absence seizures. J Neurosci 2003; 23(36): 11469-78.

[44]   Lingenhoehl K, Brom R, Heid J *et al.* Gamma-hydroxybutyrate is a weak agonist at recombinant GABA(B) receptors. Neuropharmacology 1999; 38: 1667-73.

[45]   Wu Y, Ali S, Ahmadian G *et al.* Gamma-hydroxybutyric acid (GHB) and gamma-aminobutyric acidB receptor (GABABR) binding sites are distinctive from one another: molecular evidence. Neuropharmacology 2004; 47: 1146-56.

[46]   Castelli MP, Mocci I, Pistis M *et al.* Stereoselectivity of NCS-382 binding to gamma-hydroxybutyrate receptor in the rat brain. Eur J Pharmacol 2002; 446: 1-5.

[47]   Bearden LJ, Snead OC, Healey CT, Pegram GV. Antagonism of gamma-hydroxybutyric acid-induced frequency shifts in the cortical EEG of rats by dipropylacetate. Electroencephalogr Clin Neurophysiol 1980; 49: 181-3.

[48]   Depaulis A, Bourguignon JJ, Marescaux C *et al.* Effects of gamma-hydroxybutyrate and gamma-butyrolactone derivates on spontaneous generalized non-convulsive seizures in the rat. Neuropharmacology 1988; 27: 683-9.

[49]   Crunelli V, Leresche N. Action of gamma-hydroxybutyrate on neuronal excitability and underlying membrane conductances In: Tunnicliff G, Cash CD, Eds. Gamma-hydroxybutyrate: Molecular, functional and clinical aspects. New York: Taylor and Francis 2002; pp. 75-110.

[50]   Carcak N, Aker RG, Ozdemir O, Demiralp T, Onat FY. The relationship between age-related development of spike-and-wave discharges and the resistance to amygdaloid kindling in rats with genetic absence epilepsy. Neurobiol Dis 2008; 32: 355-63.

[51]   Ryu MJ, Kim D, Kang UB *et al.* Proteomic analysis of gamma-butyrolactone-treated mouse thalamus reveals dysregulated proteins upon absence seizure. J Neurochem 2007; 102: 646-56.

[52]   Hu RQ, Cortez MA, Man HY, Wang YT, Snead OC, 3rd. Alteration of GLUR2 expression in the rat brain following absence seizures induced by gamma-hydroxybutyric acid. Epilepsy Res 2001; 44: 41-51.

[53]   Fariello RG, Golden GT. The THIP-induced model of bilateral synchronous spike and wave in rodents. Neuropharmacology 1987; 26: 161-5.

[54]   Vergnes M, Marescaux C, Micheletti G, Rumbach L, Warter JM. Blockade of "antiabsence" activity of sodium valproate by THIP in rats with petit mal-like seizures. Comparison with ethosuximide. J Neural Transm 1985; 63: 133-41.

[55]   Lundbeck. Discontinuation of development program for gaboxadol in insomnia. 2007 [03-03-2010.]; Available from: http://www.lundbeck.com/investor/Presentations/Financial_presentations/Files/Teleconference_pres/Teleconference_gaboxadol.pdf.

[56]   Smith KA, Bierkamper GG. Paradoxical role of GABA in a chronic model of petit mal (absence)-like epilepsy in the rat. Eur J Pharmacol 1990; 176: 45-55.

[57]   Persad V, Cortez MA, Snead OC, 3rd. A chronic model of atypical absence seizures: studies of developmental and gender sensitivity. Epilepsy Res 2002; 48: 111-9.

[58]   Huo JZ, Cortez MA, Snead OC, 3rd. GABA receptor proteins within lipid rafts in the AY-9944 model of atypical absence seizures. Epilepsia 2009; 50: 776-88.

[59]   Serbanescu I, Cortez MA, McKerlie C, Snead OC, 3rd. Refractory atypical absence seizures in rat: a two hit model. Epilepsy Res 2004; 62: 53-63.

[60]   Chevassus-au-Louis N, Baraban SC, Gaiarsa JL, Ben-Ari Y. Cortical malformations and epilepsy: new insights from animal models. Epilepsia 1999; 40: 811-21.

[61]   Baulac M, Pitkänen A. Research Priorities in Epilepsy for the Next Decade-A Representative View of the European Scientific Community. Epilepsia 2008.

CHAPTER 7

Kainic Acid Induced Seizures and Brain Damage: Mechanism and Relevant Therapeutic Approaches

Feng Ru Tang[1*], Koichi Kato[2*] and Weng Keong Loke[3*]

[1]*Temasek Laboratories, National University of Singapore, 5A, Engineering Drive 1, Singapore 117411;* [2]*Department of Neurosurgery, Tokyo Rosai Hospital, 4-13-21 Omoriminami, Ota-ku, Tokyo, 143-0013, Japan and* [3]*Defence Medical and Environmental Research Institute, DSO National Laboratories, 11 Stockport Road, Singapore 117605.*

Abstract: By the systemic (i.p., s.c., or i.v.) or local intracerebral injection of kainic acid (KA) into different regions of the brain of experimental animals, status epilepticus and brain damage are induced. After a latent period, progressive neuronal loss, axon sprouting and rewiring, and spontaneously recurrent seizures occurred, which are similar to the pathogenesis of the human temporal lobe epilepsy. Hence, KA models have been considered to be suitable for clarifying the mechanism of onsets of spontaneously recurrent seizures in human and for evaluating or screening anti-epileptic drugs. In this paper, we will review different seizure models induced by KA and its relevant neuropathological changes, discuss possible mechanisms for seizure generation and summarize current therapeutic approaches to control seizures and neuropathological changes. Hopefully, it will shed light on better understanding the mechanism of epiletogenesis in patients with temporal lobe epilepsy, and provide some clues for the development of novel therapeutic approaches to effectively control human intractable epilepsy.

INTRODUCTION

Kainic acid (KA) is a heterocyclic compound containing a glutamic acid backbone extracted from Kai-Nin-Sou (Digenea Simplex), which is a type of seaweed that broadly inhabits in the southern ocean of Japan, and is a hydrosoluble excitatory neuroactive amino acid. It is also one of the selective agonists for the KA type of glutamic acid receptor, which is a subtype of ion channel glutamic acid receptors. Extensive experiments from last about 30 years have well established that systemic (i.p., s.c., or i.v.) or local microinjection of KA into a specific region in the brain of experimental animals could induce status epilepticus (SE) and subsequent spontaneously recurrent seizures [1, 2, 3, 4, 5, 6, 7]. However, the mechanism of seizure generation in KA model is still not fully understood. In this paper, we will briefly introduce different seizure models induced by KA, present the relevant pathological changes and discuss about current understandings on the mechanism of seizure generations. Finally, we will summarize current therapeutic approaches to control KA- induced neuronal damage, seizures and temporal lobe epilepsy, and propose future research directions.

KAINIC-ACID INDUCED SEIZURE MODELS

Systemic (i.p., s.c., or i.v.) injections of KA

Systemic administration of the appropriate dose of kainic acid induces 'wet dog shakes', generalized tonic-clonic convulsions, teeth chattering and altered motor activity including an initial hypoactivity which transforms to a hyperactivity at later stage [8]. Neurodegeneration occurs in the pyramidal layer of CA3 area of the hippocampus and in the piriform cortex as early as 3 h following injection [8]. At this time point, a positive correlation exists between the dose of KA and the extent of the acute neurochemical changes including increases of 3,4-dihydroxyphenylacetic acid and 5-hydroxyindoleacetic acid levels and a decrease in noradrenaline levels in all brain regions investigated [9]. By 13 h to 2 weeks, neuronal somata degenerate and disappear in areas such as the olfactory cortex and parts of the amygdaloid complex, hippocampal formation, thalamus and neocortex [8]. Losses of the enzyme markers glutamic acid decarboxylase and choline acetyltransferase and incomplete parenchymal

---

*****Address correspondence to Dr. Feng-Ru Tang:** Temasek Laboratories, National University of Singapore, 5A Engineering Drive 1, #06-27, Singapore 117411. Tel: (65) 66011094; Fax: (65) 68726840; E-mail: tangfr@gmail.com. **Dr. Koichi Kato:** 4-13-21 Omoriminami, Ota-ku, Tokyo, 143-0013, Japan. Tel. 813-3742-7301; Fax. 813-3744-9310; E-mail: kkato@tokyoh.rofuku.go.jp. **Dr Weng Keong Loke:** Defense Medical and Environmental Research Institute, DSO National Laboratories, 11 Stockport Road, 20 Science Park Drive, Singapore 117605. Tel: (65)68712885; Fax: (65)68730742; E-mail: lwengkeo@dso.org.sg

necrosis and haemorrhages occur in the hippocampus, amygdala, entorhinal and pyriform cortex, and olfactory bulb in animals which have undergone severe convulsions [2, 9]. In the rat hippocampal formation after intravenous KA injection, degeneration of CA4-derived afferent fibers provokes the growth of mossy fiber collaterals into the fascia dentata. These aberrant fibers form granule cell-granule cell synapses, which have been suggested to be involved in seizure generation [10]. Following intraperitoneal kainic acid injection an extensive axonal sprouting of CA1 pyramidal neurons, with many axonal branches entering the pyramidal cell layer and stratum radiatum, regions that are not innervated by axonal collaterals of CA1 pyramidal neurons in control animals also occurs. Concurrently with this anatomical reorganization, a large increase of the spontaneous glutamatergic drive is observed in the dendrites and somata of CA1 pyramidal cells. Furthermore, electrical activation of the reorganized CA1 associational pathway evokes epileptiform bursts in CA1 pyramidal cells, suggesting that reactive plasticity could contribute to the hyperexcitability of CA1 pyramidal neurons and to the propagation of seizures [11]. Subcutaneous injection of KA induces neurodegeneration in the hippocampal CA1, CA3 areas, the dentate hilar regions, amygdaloid and thalamic nuclei; and frontoparietotemporal, entorhinal and piriform cortices 3 days after KA administration. Degeneration severity peaks at 6 days and decreases progressively until 168 days after KA injection [12]. Aberrant mossy fiber sprouting is present in the inner molecular layer of dentate gyrus as early as 6 days after KA injection. Microgliosis and astrogliosis peaks at 28 days and are generally colocalized with the distribution of neuronal degeneration [12].

In immature rat (postnatal day 15) after KA injection, retrograde tracing experiments show a larger dorsoventral extent of retrograde labeling in the CA1 pyramidal region after tracer injections in subiculum. The synaptic reorganization of the CA1 projection to subiculum is noted in the absence of overt neuronal injury in subiculum or CA1. In contrast, mossy fiber sprouting is detected into the stratum oriens of CA3 with limited neuronal injury to CA3 pyramidal neurons. No mossy fiber sprouting into the inner molecular layer of the dentate gyrus, or CA1 sprouting into the stratum moleculare of CA1 are demonstrated, suggesting that morphological plasticity in the immature brain appears more extensive in distal, but not proximal, projections of hippocampal pathways, and across hippocampal lamellae, and the abnormal connectivity between hippocampal lamellae may play a role in the increased susceptibility to injury and hyperexcitability associated with later convulsive insults [13].

Seizure Models Induced by Intracerebral Injections of KA

Intra-Amygdala Injection

Unilateral intra-amygdaloid application of low doses of KA elicits generalized convulsive seizures which often culminate in fatal SE rapidly. Spontaneous recurrent seizures are observed for several hours starting approximately 10 min after the application of KA [14]. By 2 to 3 weeks after KA injection, 64% of rats developed spontaneous limbic seizures [15]. When KA is injected into the cat amygdala, focal SE in the limbic system is observed for 3 days. Secondary epileptogenic foci are then established in the contralateral amygdala, and amygdaloid seizures begin to occur alternatively on both sides and finally trigger frequent limbic seizures from 3 to 5 weeks after KA injection. Spontaneous secondarily generalized seizures develop about 4 weeks after KA injection and occur once or twice a week thereafter [16]. Pathologically, focal necrosis with perifocal gliosis occurs at the injection site of the amygdala. Ipsilateral pyriform cortex is also affected. Neuronal loss, gliosis and atrophy are mainly in the CA3 pyramidal layer of the ipsilateral side of the hippocampus [15, 16].

Intra-Hippocampus Injection

Intrahippocampal injections of KA induced epileptiform behavior accompanied with a rapid and complete degeneration of neuronal perikarya, gliosis and atrophy in the entire hippocampal formation [17]. The activity of the biochemical markers for GABAergic neurons including glutamic acid decarboxylase, endogenous GABA and synaptosomal uptake of [3H]GABA is decreased by almost 50%. The extrinsic hippocampal cholinergic and noradrenergic afferents also exhibit significant alteration. The specific activity of tyrosine hydroxylase is significantly increased in the injected hippocampus, the synaptosomal high affinity uptake process for [3H]choline and [3H]norepinephrine are significantly reduced at 10 days after injection. Whereas the level of endogenous acetylcholine is elevated in the lesioned hippocampus at 2 days after injection, the level of endogenous norepinephrine is reduced [18]. Glutamate decarboxylase immunoreactivity (GAD-IR) puncta are significantly increased in the ipsi- and contralateral inner molecular layers (IML) of the dentate gyrus when compared to sham or normal controls. KA lesion also induces mossy fiber recurrent collateral sprouting into the ipsi- and contralateral dentate gyrus IMLs. The loss of both the commissural and ipsilateral associational afferents to the dentate gyrus apparently induces sprouting into their ipsi- and contralateral termination zones by granule cell mossy fibers and GAD-IR axons, thus establishing an abnormal circuitry near the observed pathology in the KA model of epilepsy [19]. Sprouting of local axon collaterals of CA1 pyramidal cells in stratum oriens and in the alveus also occurs. This local increase in axon collaterals may contribute to the epileptiform activity in the CA1 area by providing recurrent excitation *via* newly formed synaptic contacts with pyramidal cell dendrites [20].

Intra-Thalamus Injection

When KA is injected unilaterally into the posterolateral ventral nuclei (VPL) of the thalamus, multiple spikes are observed in the VPL, which propagate to the subcortical structures, and then bilaterally to the cortex. About 3-4 h after the injection, small spike and wave complexes repeatedly appear for a short period of time in cortical leads and cats exhibit behavioral arrest with unresponsiveness during the seizures. About 24 h after the injection, generalized small spike and wave complexes are observed intermittently in cortical and subcortical structures. They persist for 4-5s and are associated with behavioral arrest and staring, suggesting that a unilateral microinjection of KA into VPL induces petit mal-like seizure, and VPL plays an important role in the generation or transfer of spike and wave complexes [21]. Histological examination reveals very circumscribed neuronal cell loss and pyknosis in the left VPL where kainic acid is injected.

Intra-thalamus injection of KA into the left mediodorsal nucleus (MD) of Wistar rats induces bilateral synchronous spike and wave complexes appear at 2 hours after injection. The waveforms continue for about 5-7 hours in the bilateral MDs, ipsilateral sensorimotor cortex, and basolateral nucleus of the amygdala. The associated behavioral changes are mainly those of behavioral arrest and staring, associated with occasional limbic seizures. Clear metabolic increases are found in the ipsilateral frontal cortex, hippocampus, and amygdale suggesting that MD is involved in both the mechanism of spike and wave complexes in the bilateral frontal cortices, and in seizure propagation to the limbic system [22]. Pathologically, small gliotic lesions, pyknosis and neuronal loss are observed in the injection site. Loss of pyramidal neurons in the CA3 and CA4 areas of the ipsilateral hippocampus also occurs.

Intra-Striatal Injection

After intrastriatal injection of KA, neuronal degeneration spread unevenly into contiguous structures from the injected site and affects the ipsilateral pyriform cortex and amygdala, the deep layers of the overlying cerebral cortex, and the medial aspects of the bed nucleus of the stria terminalis and of the nucleus accumbens. The pyriform cortex contralateral to the side of injection also undergoes degeneration. A subpopulation of pyramidal cells in layer IV of the lateral neocortex and the CA3-CA4 pyramidal cells in the ipsilateral hippocampus are selectively affected, whereas adjacent neurons remain intact. The distribution of agyrophilic fibers and terminals in subcortical structures is consistent with the degeneration of neurons of origin in the affected striatal and extrastriatal regions. An intense astrocytic response in all areas affected by acute neuronal degeneration also occurs [23].

When KA is injected into the left globus pallidus pars externa, it evokes not only epileptic excitation of the cortex but also transient enhancement of the globus pallidus-substantia nigra circuit. Histopathological study reveals a small gliotic lesion with neuronal cell loss around the cannula tip. Neither degeneration nor neuronal cell loss in the ipsilateral hippocampus are observed. The autoradiogram using [14C]2-deoxyglucose during seizure status demonstrates a remarkable increase of local cerebral glucose utilization not only in the globus pallidus pars externa but also in the globus pallidus interna. An increase glucose metabolism is also found in the medial and lateral septal nucleus, substantia nigra, hippocampus, frontal cortex, parietal cortex, piriform cortex, entorhinal cortex, accumbens nucleus, ventral and lateral nucleus of the thalamus, amygdala, and ventral nucleus of hypothalamus [24].

Intra-Midbrain Injection

Injection of KA into the substantia nigra pars reticulata has been shown to induce a secondary generalized seizure status. Limbic seizure manifestations such as salivation are observed as an initial symptom and followed by rolling and generalized tonic seizures. [(14)C]deoxyglucose autoradiographic study demonstrates increased local cerebral glucose metabolism in the medial and lateral septal nucleus, substantia nigra, hippocampus, parietal cortex, piriform cortex, medial and lateral geniculate nucleus, anterodorsal, lateral and ventral nucleus of the thalamus, amygdala and midbrain reticular formation, suggesting that the decreased function of the GABAergic projection system induced by an excessive epileptic excitation of substantia nigra pars reticulata may play an important role in the secondary generalization [25]. Focal electrical seizures are induced when injection of KA into a unilateral mesencephalic reticular formation in cats and rats. The initial clinical change during each seizure is behavioral arrest. These seizures immediately develop to generalized seizures, which are characterized by generalized tonic convulsions with short-term clonic convulsions. High glucose utilization is observed in the MRF, bilateral thalamus, forebrain and bilateral cerebral cortices, suggesting an active participation of MRF in the mechanism of generalized seizures [26-27]. When injected into the raphe dorsal nucleus of cats, the enhancement of brain excitability level up to hyperexcitation (seizures) is observed. Histopathological study shows a dose-dependent cytoarchitectural disorganization at the injection site and in many other brain structures, suggesting that the hyperexcitatory effect of KA on brain excitability may be due to its excitatory action, which triggers neuronal hyperactivity in neural circuits connected with the raphe dorsal nucleus [28-30].

Intra-Cerebraventricular Injection of KA

It has been well documented that intraventricular KA injection induces neuronal damage in CA4, CA3 and CA1 areas of the hippocampus and in the hilus of the dentate gyrus [31-32] and mossy fiber sprouting [10]. In the mossy fiber system, enkephalin immunoreactivity (ENK-I) is dramatically elevated, dynorphin immunoreactivity is reduced, and CCK immunoreactivity (CCK-I) is either severely reduced or completely absent [33]. In the dentate gyrus, granule cell neurogenesis is increased bilaterally 1 week after a single unilateral intracerebroventricular injection of KA [34].

MECHANISMS OF KA INDUCED BRAIN DAMAGES, AND SEIZURE GENERATION

Early studies have suggested that KA induced damage in the injection site may be caused by its direct stimulation of the postsynaptic receptor, its indirect destruction by accentuating the toxicity of endogenous glutamic acid *via* release of glutamate or inhibition of high affinity glutamate uptake or by its toxic metabolite [35-37]. At sites remote from the site of injection, the damage may be due to its intra-axonal transportation and releasing at the axon terminals, transneuronal or retrograde degenerative effects secondary to destruction of neurons at the injection site, transmitting or at least enhancing by intense electrical activity in axons emanating from the injection site [8]. However, Krespan *et al.* (1982) indicate that the glutamate released by KA comes from nonsynaptic instead of synaptic pools [38]. This is in agreement with later study showing that the ability of KA to release amino acids plays no significant role in its neurotoxic effects [39]. Fuller and Olney (1981) find that a seizure mechanism underlies the limbic brain damage induced by systemic KA may have two mutually reinforcing components--a glutamergic excitatory component and a GABAergic disinhibitory component as pretreatment with 2 anticonvulsants (diazepam or phenobarbital) markedly reduces both the seizure and brain damaging actions of KA [40]. Ligand binding studies reveal specific receptors for KA, suggesting that it may directly act on its own receptors to cause neurotoxic effects [41]. This is confirmed by the cloning of KA receptor subunits [42-45]. Further study demonstrates that KA receptor activation can induce transcription-independent apoptosis in neurons [46]. KA could also induce neuronal swelling by a sodium- and chloride-dependent mechanism, and the enhancement of swelling in low calcium is due to an increased sodium uptake [47]. Combined with recent study showing that GluR5 KA receptor has a unique role in triggering epileptiform activity in the amygdala and could participate in long-term plasticity mechanisms that underlie epileptogenesis [48], it strongly suggests that KA receptors may be main targets of KA to produce the epileptogenic and excitotoxic effects and for the development of antiepileptic drugs and neuroprotective agents [7]. Mossy fiber sprouting has been considered to be involved in epileptogenesis in KA model [10]. However, blockade of KA-induced mossy fiber sprouting by cycloheximide does not prevent epileptogenesis in rats [49-50]. Subsequent studies indicate that mossy fiber sprouting is a consequence rather than the cause of the hyperexcitable hippocampal network resulting from KA induced seizures [51]. Whether sprouting of local axon collaterals in other brain regions such as CA1 area is involved in the generation of spontaneously recurrent seizures remains to be further investigated [19, 20]. Recent studies in intra-hippocampal KA injection model show that prolonged seizures prompt NO-, O(2)(-)-, and peroxynitrite-dependent reduction in mitochondrial respiratory enzyme Complex I activity, leading to cytochrome c/caspase-3-dependent apoptotic cell death in the hippocampal CA3 subfield [52] and upregulation of nitric oxide synthase II by nuclear factor-kappaB also promotes apoptotic neuronal cell death in the hippocampus

[53], these findings are in agreement with many of previous reports [54-57], and suggests that reactive oxygen species may be involved in KA-induced brain damage and seizure activities, and are potential therapeutic target for prevention of KA–induced neuronal loss and epileptogenesis.

THERAPEUTIC APPROACHES

Many different drugs have been tested in KA models to prevent brain damage, seizures and epileptogenesis. Pretreatment with anticonvulsants such as diazepam, phenobarbital or levetiracetam markedly reduces both the seizure and brain damaging induced by KA, whereas, phenytoin or valproic acid fail to suppress either phenomenon [58-59]. Mannitol treatment prevents propagation of seizures and brain damage in the KA model of epilepsy by washing out brain oedema [60].

However, NMDA antagonists such as ketamine, phencyclidine, and MK-801 could only prevent seizure-related brain damage without suppressing seizure activity [61]. Growth factors such as basic fibroblast growth factor (bFGF) [62-63], acidic fibroblast growth factor (aFGF) [64], brain-derived neurotrophic factor [65-66] have also been shown to prevent seizure-associated brain damage, but not seizure generation. Low dose administration using encapsulated BDNF-secreting cells exerts neuroprotective effects with enhanced neurogenesis on KA model of epilepsy [66]. EUK-134, a synthetic superoxide dismutase/catalase mimetic, could not control KA-induced seizure activity, but could produce a highly significant reduction in increased protein nitration, activator protein-1- and NF-kappaB-binding activity and spectrin proteolysis as well as in neuronal damage resulting from seizure activity in limbic structures [67]. It further supports the argument that reactive oxygen species are involved in KA-induced brain damage [52, 54-57].

Melatonin may exert its protective property by inhibiting polyamine responses [68], activating plasma membrane receptors and PI3K-Akt signaling pathway in astrocytes [69], decreasing hippocampal lipid peroxidation (LPO) and increasing Coenzyme Q10 (CoQ 10) [70] or scavenging of hydroxyl radicals [71]. Budziszewska *et al.* (2001) indicate that estrone attenuates KA-induced seizures, mortality and excitotoxicity in male mice. The suppressive effect of estrone on clonic seizures may involve intracellular receptors, whereas its antineurotoxic activity seems to depend on a non-genomic mechanism [72]. Metallothionein reduces central nervous system inflammation, neurodegeneration, and cell death following KA-induced epileptic seizures by indirect anti-inflammatory and antioxidant actions and direct effects on the neurons [73]. The Rb1 and Rb3 ginsenosides from a partial purification of the whole Ginseng extract has significant anticonvulsant properties. However, Ginseng extract made from either the root or leaves/stems was ineffective against KA induced seizures [74].

Phospholipase A(2) inhibitors, quinacrine and chloroquine, arachidonyl trifluoromethyl ketone, bromoenol lactone, cytidine 5-diphosphoamines, and vitamin E, not only inhibit phospholipase A(2) activity but also prevent KA-induced neurodegeneration, suggesting that phospholipase A(2) is involved in the neurodegenerative process. It also suggests that phospholipase A(2) inhibitors can be used as neuroprotectants and anti-inflammatory agents against neurodegenerative processes in neurodegenerative diseases [75].

Manganese complexes of curcumin (Cp-Mn) and diacetylcurcumin (DiAc-Cp-Mn) could suppress KA-induced neuronal injury marker expression, and may be effective in treatment of excitotoxicity-induced neurodegenerative diseases [76]. Chelatable iron is an important catalyst for the initiation and propagation of free radical reactions and implicated in the pathogenesis of diverse neuronal disorders. Liang *et al.* (2008) recently indicate that systemically administered N,N'-bis (2-hydroxybenzyl) ethylenediamine-N,N'-diacetic acid (HBED), a synthetic iron chelator, ameliorates SE-induced changes in chelatable iron, mitochondrial oxidative stress (8-hydroxy-2' deoxyguanosine and glutathione depletion), mitochondrial DNA integrity and hippocampal cell loss, suggesting a role for mitochondrial iron in the pathogenesis of SE-induced brain damage and subcellular iron chelation as a novel therapeutic approach for its management [77]. Persistent zinc depletion in the mossy fiber terminals by continuous injection of midazolam (MDZ) could also suppress seizure generation [78].

Intraperitoneal taurine injection has been proven to reduce or completely stop seizure activity and exert neuroprotective actions [79]. Resveratrol, a phytoalexin which has multi- functional effects such as neuroprotection, anti-inflammatory and anti-cancer, has recently been shown to be a potent anti-epilepsy agent, which protects against epileptogenesis and progression of the KA-induced temporal lobe epilepsy [80]. β(2)-adrenoceptor agonist clenbuterol ameliorates KA-induced apoptosis, reduces inflammatory cytokine expression, and expression of inducible nitric oxide synthase (iNOS), indolamine 2,3-dioxygenase (IDO) and kynurenine monooxygenase (KMO) and CD11b, and increases BDNF and NGF expression in KA-treated rats, and has anti-inflammatory and neurotrophic actions and elicits a neuroprotective effect in the KA model of neurodegeneration [81]. Inhibitors for fatty acid amide hydrolase (FAAH), the enzyme responsible for metabolism of the endocannabinoid anandamide, such as AM5206 [82] and URB597 [83] could not only reduce seizure activity, but also prevent cytoskeletal damage and synaptic protein decline.

Experimental increase of CB1 cannabinoid receptor gene dosage in principal neurons has also been reported to reduce KA-induced seizure severity and mortality, and has therapeutic effects in KA-induced hippocampal pathogenesis [84]. Das *et al.* (2010) recently demonstrate that the anti-epileptic drugs that block both Na(+) channels and Ca(2+) channels (Valproic Acid and Zonisamide) are significantly more effective than agents that block only Na(+) channels (Lamotrigine, Rufinamide, and Oxcarbazepine) for attenuating seizure-induced hippocampal neurodegeneration [85]. The mammalian target of rapamycin (mTOR) inhibitor rapamycin blocks both the acute and chronic phases of seizure-induced mTOR activation and decreases KA-induced neuronal cell death, neurogenesis, mossy fiber sprouting, and the development of spontaneous epilepsy when administered before KA injection. The chronic phase of mTOR activation, mossy fiber sprouting and epilepsy are also prevented when rapamycin is given after KA-induced SE. It strongly suggested that mTOR signaling mediates mechanisms of epileptogenesis in the KA rat model and that mTOR inhibitors have potential antiepileptogenic effects in this model [86].

CONCLUSION

KA- induced animal models of status epilepticus and temporal lobe epilepsy have been well established since the later 1970's. However, the mechanism of KA- induced brain damage and epileptogenesis is still not clear, this may be due to the fact that most of the previous studies have focused on NMDA and AMPA receptors or other neurotransmitters and their receptors before the cloning of KA receptor subunits. Therefore, the proposed mechanism of brain damage, seizure generation and epileptogenesis, and the therapeutic effect in previous studies may not be the direct actions of KA. The failing of clinical trial of NMDA antagonists in controlling of seizures and prevention of epileptogenesis has now spurred a new surge of research on the roles of KA receptor subunits in neurodegenerative disorders including temporal lobe epilepsy. Given the fact that KA receptor subunits appear to be primary targets of KA in the KA models, systemic study of the roles of different subunits of KA receptors in brain damage and epileptogenesis may provide new clues for better understanding the mechanism of epileptogenesis in patients with temporal lobe epilepsy, and for screening drugs targeting on KA receptor system to effectively control intractable epilepsy.

REFERENCES

[1]   Nadler JV. Minireview. Kainic acid as a tool for the study of temporal lobe epilepsy. Life Sci 1981; 29: 2031-42.
[2]   Ben-Ari Y, Tremblay E, Ottersen OP, Naquet R. Evidence suggesting secondary epileptogenic lesions after kainic acid: pretreatment with diazepam reduces distant but not local brain damage. Brain Res 1979; 165: 362-365.
[3]   Treiman DM, Walton NY, Kendrick C. A progressive sequence of electroencephalographic changes during generalized convulsive status epilepticus. Epilepsy Res 1990; 5: 49-60.
[4]   Tanaka T, Tanaka S, Fujita T, Takano K, Fukuda H, Sako K, Yonemasu Y. Experimental complex partial seizures induced by a microinjection of kainic acid into limbic structures. Prog Neurobiol 1992; 38: 317-334.
[5]   Ben-Ari Y, Cossart R. Kainate, a double agent that generates seizures: two decades of progress. Trends Neurosci 2000; 23: 580-7.
[6]   Leite JP, Garcia-Cairasco N, Cavalheiro EA. New insights from the use of pilocarpine and kainate models. Epilepsy Res 2002; 50: 93-103.
[7]   Vincent P, Mulle C. Kainate receptors in epilepsy and excitotoxicity. Neuroscience 2009; 158: 309-23.
[8]   Schwob JE, Fuller T, Price JL, Olney JW. Widespread patterns of neuronal damage following systemic or intracerebral injections of kainic acid: a histological study. Neuroscience 1980; 5: 991-1014.
[9]   Sperk G, Lassmann H, Baran H, Seitelberger F, Hornykiewicz O. Kainic acid-induced seizures: dose-relationship of behavioural, neurochemical and histopathological changes. Brain Res 1985; 338: 289-95.

[10]   Tauck DL, Nadler JV. Evidence of functional mossy fiber sprouting in hippocampal formation of kainic acid-treated rats. J Neurosci 1985; 5:1016-22.

[11]   Esclapez M, Hirsch JC, Ben-Ari Y, Bernard C. Newly formed excitatory pathways provide a substrate for hyperexcitability in experimental temporal lobe epilepsy. J Comp Neurol 1999; 408: 449-60.

[12]   Sharma AK, Jordan WH, Reams RY, Hall DG, Snyder PW. Temporal profile of clinical signs and histopathologic changes in an F-344 rat model of kainic acid-induced mesial temporal lobe epilepsy. Toxicol Pathol 2008; 36: 932-43.

[13]   Cross DJ, Cavazos JE. Synaptic reorganization in subiculum and CA3 after early-life status epilepticus in the kainic acid rat model. Epilepsy Res 2007; 73: 156-65.

[14]   Ben-Ari Y, Lagowska J. Epileptogenic action of intra-amygdaloid injection of kainic acid. C R Acad Sci Hebd Seances Acad Sci D 1978; 287: 813-6.

[15]   Tanaka S, Kondo S, Tanaka T, Yonemasu Y. Long-term observation of rats after unilateral intra-amygdaloid injection of kainic acid. Brain Res 1988; 463: 163-7.

[16]   Tanaka T, Kaijima M, Yonemasu Y, Cepeda C. Spontaneous secondarily generalized seizures induced by a single microinjection of kainic acid into unilateral amygdala in cats. Electroencephalogr Clin Neurophysiol 1985; 61: 422-9.

[17]   Schwarcz R, Zaczek R, Coyle JT. Microinjection of kainic acid into the rat hippocampus. Eur J Pharmacol 1978; 50: 209-20.

[18]   Zaczek R, Nelson MF, Coyle JT. Effects of anaesthetics and anticonvulsants on the action of kainic acid in the rat hippocampus. Eur J Pharmacol 1978; 52: 323-7.

[19]   Davenport CJ, Brown WJ, Babb TL. Sprouting of GABAergic and mossy fiber axons in dentate gyrus following intrahippocampal kainate in the rat. Exp Neurol 1990; 109: 180-90.

[20]   Perez Y, Morin F, Beaulieu C, Lacaille JC. Axonal sprouting of CA1 pyramidal cells in hyperexcitable hippocampal slices of kainate-treated rats. Eur J Neurosci 1996; 8: 736-748.

[21]   Araki T, Tanaka T, Tanaka S, Yonemasu Y, Kato M, Goto I. Kainic acid-induced thalamic seizure in cats--a possible model of petit mal seizure. Epilepsy Res 1992; 13: 223-9.

[22]   Kato K, Urino T, Hori T *et al.* Experimental petit mal-like seizure induced by microinjection of kainic acid into the unilateral mediodorsal nucleus of the thalamus. Neurol Med Chir (Tokyo) 2008; 48: 285-90.

[23]   Zaczek R, Simonton S, Coyle JT. Local and distant neuronal degeneration following intrastriatal injection of kainic acid. J Neuropathol Exp Neurol 1980; 39: 245-64.

[24]   Sawamura A, Hashizume K, Tanaka T. Electrophysiological, behavioral and metabolical features of globus pallidus seizures induced by a microinjection of kainic acid in rats. Brain Res 2002: 935: 1-8.

[25]   Sawamura A, Hashizume K, Yoshida K, Tanaka T. Kainic acid-induced substantia nigra seizure in rats: behavior, EEG and metabolism. Brain Res 2001; 911: 89-95.

[26]   Tanaka T, Fujita T, Tanaka S, Araki T, Yonemasu Y. Secondary generalization in kainic acid-induced focal seizures in unanesthetized cats. Jpn J Psychiatry Neurol 1991; 45: 243-8.

[27]   Hashizume K, Tanaka T, Fujita T, Tanaka S. Generalized seizures induced by an epileptic focus in the mesencephalic reticular formation: impact on the understanding of the generalizing mechanism. Stereotact Funct Neurosurg 2000; 74: 153-60.

[28]   Moyanova S, Rousseva S, Ivanova A, Dimov S. Intraraphedorsal kainic acid induces paroxysmal electroencephalographic changes in some brain structures of cats. Exp Neurol 1986; 93: 98-109.

[29]   Moyanova S, Rousseva S, Dimov S. Changes in the EEG-reactions to repetitive peripheral and central electrical stimulation by intraraphedorsal kainic acid in the cat. Methods Find Exp Clin Pharmacol 1987; 9: 39-47.

[30]   Moyanova S, Riche D. Injections of kainic acid into the raphe dorsal nucleus in freely moving cats: electroencephalographic, behavioral and histopathological consequences. Methods Find Exp Clin Pharmacol 1992; 14: 49-60.

[31]   Nadler JV, Perry BW, Cotman CW. Intraventricular kainic acid preferentially destroys hippocampal pyramidal cells. Nature 1978; 271: 676-7.

[32]   Franck JE. Dynamic alterations in hippocampal morphology following intra-ventricular kainic acid. Acta Neuropathol 1984; 62: 242-53.

[33]   Gall C. Seizures induce dramatic and distinctly different changes in enkephalin, dynorphin, and CCK immunoreactivities in mouse hippocampal mossy fibers. J Neurosci 1988; 8: 1852-62.

[34]   Gray WP, Sundstrom LE. Kainic acid increases the proliferation of granule cell progenitors in the dentate gyrus of the adult rat. Brain Res 1998; 790: 52-9.

[35]   McGeer EG, McGeer PL, Singh K. Kainate-induced degeneration of neostriatal neurons: dependency upon corticostriatal tract. Brain Res 1978; 139: 381-3.

[36] Ferkany JW, Zaczek R, Coyle JT. Kainic acid stimulates excitatory amino acid neurotransmitter release at presynaptic receptors. Nature 1982; 298:757-9.

[37] Ferkany JW, Zaczek R, Coyle JT. The mechanism of kainic acid neurotoxicity. Nature 1984; 308: 561-2.

[38] Krespan B, Berl S, Nicklas WJ. Alteration in neuronal-glial metabolism of glutamate by the neurotoxin kainic acid. J Neurochem 1982; 38: 509-18.

[39] Garthwaite J, Garthwaite G. The mechanism of kainic acid neurotoxicity. Nature 1983; 305:138-40.

[40] Fuller TA, Olney JW. Only certain anticonvulsants protect against kainate neurotoxicity. Neurobehav Toxicol Teratol 1981; 3: 355-61.

[41] Coyle JT, Ferkany JW, Zaczek R. Kainic acid: insights from a neurotoxin into the pathophysiology of Huntington's disease. Neurobehav Toxicol Teratol 1983; 5: 617-24.

[42] Hollmann M, O'Shea-Greenfield A, Rogers SW, Heinemann S. Cloning by functional expression of a member of the glutamate receptor family. Nature 1989; 342: 643-8.

[43] Boulter J, Hollmann M, O'Shea-Greenfield A, Hartley M, Deneris E, Maron C, Heinemann S. Molecular cloning and functional expression of glutamate receptor subunit genes. Science 1990; 249: 1033-7.

[44] Hollmann M, Heinemann S. Cloned glutamate receptors. Annu Rev Neurosci 1994; 17:31–108.

[45] Bettler B, Mulle C. Review: neurotransmitter receptors. II. AMPA and kainate receptors. Neuropharmacology 1995; 34: 123–139.

[46] Simonian NA, Getz RL, Leveque JC, Konradi C, Coyle JT. Kainic acid induces apoptosis in neurons. Neuroscience 1996; 75: 1047-55.

[47] Berdichevsky E, Muñoz C, Riveros N, Cartier L, Orrego F. Neuropathological changes in the rat brain cortex *in vitro*: effects of kainic acid and of ion substitutions. Brain Res 1987; 423: 213-20.

[48] Rogawski MA, Gryder D, Castaneda D, Yonekawa W, Banks MK, Lia H. GluR5 kainate receptors, seizures, and the amygdala. Ann N Y Acad Sci 2003; 985:150-62.

[49] Longo BM, Mello LE. Blockade of pilocarpine- or kainate-induced mossy fiber sprouting by cycloheximide does not prevent subsequent epileptogenesis in rats. Neurosci Lett 1997; 226: 163-6.

[50] Longo BM, Mello LE. Supragranular mossy fiber sprouting is not necessary for spontaneous seizures in the intrahippocampal kainate model of epilepsy in the rat. Epilepsy Res 1998; 32: 172-82.

[51] Bender RA, Dubé C, Gonzalez-Vega R, Mina EW, Baram TZ. Mossy fiber plasticity and enhanced hippocampal excitability, without hippocampal cell loss or altered neurogenesis, in an animal model of prolonged febrile seizures. Hippocampus 2003;13: 399-412.

[52] Chuang YC, Chen SD, Liou CW *et al.* Contribution of nitric oxide, superoxide anion, and peroxynitrite to activation of mitochondrial apoptotic signaling in hippocampal CA3 subfield following experimental temporal lobe status epilepticus. Epilepsia 2009; 50: 731-46.

[53] Chuang YC, Chen SD, Lin TK *et al.* Transcriptional upregulation of nitric oxide synthase II by nuclear factor-kappaB promotes apoptotic neuronal cell death in the hippocampus following experimental status epilepticus. J Neurosci Res 2010; 88: 1898-907.

[54] Layton ME, Pazdernik TL. Reactive oxidant species in piriform cortex extracellular fluid during seizures induced by systemic kainic acid in rats. J Mol Neurosci 1999; 13: 63-8.

[55] Liang LP, Ho YS, Patel M. Mitochondrial superoxide production in kainate-induced hippocampal damage. Neuroscience 2000; 101: 563-70.

[56] Liang LP, Patel M. Mitochondrial oxidative stress and increased seizure susceptibility in Sod2(-/+) mice. Free Radic Biol Med 2004; 36: 542-54.

[57] Milatovic D, Gupta RC, Dettbarn WD. Involvement of nitric oxide in kainic acid-induced excitotoxicity in rat brain. Brain Res 2002; 957: 330-7.

[58] Fuller TA, Olney JW. Only certain anticonvulsants protect against kainate neurotoxicity. Neurobehav Toxicol Teratol 1981; 3: 355-61.

[59] Marini H, Costa C, Passaniti M *et al.* Levetiracetam protects against kainic acid-induced toxicity. Life Sci 2004; 74: 1253-64.

[60] Baran H, Lassmann H, Sperk G, Seitelberger F, Hornykiewicz O. Effect of mannitol treatment on brain neurotransmitter markers in kainic acid-induced epilepsy. Neuroscience 1987; 21: 679-84.

[61] Clifford DB, Olney JW, Benz AM, Fuller TA, Zorumski CF. Ketamine, phencyclidine, and MK-801 protect against kainic acid-induced seizure-related brain damage. Epilepsia 1990; 31: 382-90.

[62] Liu Z, D'Amore PA, Mikati M, Gatt A, Holmes GL. Neuroprotective effect of chronic infusion of basic fibroblast growth factor on seizure-associated hippocampal damage. Brain Res 1993; 626: 335-8.

[63]   Liu Z, Holmes GL. Basic fibroblast growth factor is highly neuroprotective against seizure-induced long-term behavioural deficits. Neuroscience 1997; 76: 1129-38.

[64]   Cuevas P, Revilla C, Herreras O, Largo C, Giménez-Gallego G. Neuroprotective effect of acidic fibroblast growth factor on seizure-associated brain damage. Neurol Res 1994; 16: 365-9.

[65]   Tandon P, Yang Y, Das K, Holmes GL, Stafstrom CE. Neuroprotective effects of brain-derived neurotrophic factor in seizures during development. Neuroscience 1999; 91: 293-303.

[66]   Kuramoto S, Yasuhara T, Agari T *et al.* BDNF-secreting capsule exerts neuroprotective effects on epilepsy model of rats. Brain Res 2011; 1368: 281-9.

[67]   Rong Y, Doctrow SR, Tocco G, Baudry M. EUK-134, a synthetic superoxide dismutase and catalase mimetic, prevents oxidative stress and attenuates kainate-induced neuropathology. Proc Natl Acad Sci 1999; 96: 9897-902.

[68]   Lee YK, Lee SR, Kim CY. Melatonin attenuates the changes in polyamine levels induced by systemic kainate administration in rat brains. J Neurol Sci 2000; 178: 124-31.

[69]   Kong PJ, Byun JS, Lim SY *et al.* Melatonin Induces Akt Phosphorylation through Melatonin Receptor- and PI3K-Dependent Pathways in Primary Astrocytes. Korean J Physiol Pharmacol 2008; 12: 37-41.

[70]   Yalcin A, Kilinc E, Kocturk S, Resmi H, Sozmen EY. Effect of melatonin cotreatment against kainic acid on coenzyme Q10, lipid peroxidation and Trx mRNA in rat hippocampus. Int J Neurosci 2004; 114: 1085-97.

[71]   Mohanan PV, Yamamoto HA. Preventive effect of melatonin against brain mitochondria DNA damage, lipid peroxidation and seizures induced by kainic acid. Toxicol Lett 2002; 129: 99-105.

[72]   Budziszewska B, Leśkiewicz M, Kubera M, Jaworska-Feil L, Kajta M, Lasoń W. Estrone, but not 17 beta-estradiol, attenuates kainate-induced seizures and toxicity in male mice. Exp Clin Endocrinol Diabetes 2001; 109: 168-73.

[73]   Penkowa M, Florit S, Giralt M *et al.* Metallothionein reduces central nervous system inflammation, neurodegeneration, and cell death following kainic acid-induced epileptic seizures. J Neurosci Res 2005; 79: 522-34.

[74]   Lian XY, Zhang ZZ, Stringer JL. Anticonvulsant activity of ginseng on seizures induced by chemical convulsants. Epilepsia 2005; 46: 15-22.

[75]   Farooqui AA, Ong WY, Horrocks LA. Inhibitors of brain phospholipase A2 activity: their neuropharmacological effects and therapeutic importance for the treatment of neurologic disorders. Pharmacol Rev 2006; 58: 591-620.

[76]   Sumanont Y, Murakami Y, Tohda M, Vajragupta O, Watanabe H, Matsumoto K. Effects of manganese complexes of curcumin and diacetylcurcumin on kainic acid-induced neurotoxic responses in the rat hippocampus. Biol Pharm Bull 2007; 30:1732-9.

[77]   Liang LP, Jarrett SG, Patel M. Chelation of mitochondrial iron prevents seizure-induced mitochondrial dysfunction and neuronal injury. J Neurosci 2008; 28: 11550-6.

[78]   Mitsuya K, Nitta N, Suzuki F. Persistent zinc depletion in the mossy fiber terminals in the intrahippocampal kainate mouse model of mesial temporal lobe epilepsy. Epilepsia 2009; 50:1979-90.

[79]   Junyent F, Utrera J, Romero R *et al.* Prevention of epilepsy by taurine treatments in mice experimental model. J Neurosci Res 2009; 87: 1500-8.

[80]   Wu Z, Xu Q, Zhang L, Kong D, Ma R, Wang L. Protective effect of resveratrol against kainate-induced temporal lobe epilepsy in rats. Neurochem Res 2009; 34: 1393-400.

[81]   Gleeson LC, Ryan KJ, Griffin EW, Connor TJ, Harkin A. The β2-adrenoceptor agonist clenbuterol elicits neuroprotective, anti-inflammatory and neurotrophic actions in the kainic acid model of excitotoxicity. Brain Behav Immun 2010; 24: 1354-61.

[82]   Naidoo V, Nikas SP, Karanian DA *et al.* A new generation fatty acid amide hydrolase inhibitor protects against kainate-induced excitotoxicity. J Mol Neurosci 2011; 43: 493-502.

[83]   Coomber B, O'Donoghue MF, Mason R. Inhibition of endocannabinoid metabolism attenuates enhanced hippocampal neuronal activity induced by kainic acid. Synapse 2008; 62: 746-55.

[84]   Guggenhuber S, Monory K, Lutz B, Klugmann M. AAV vector-mediated overexpression of CB1 cannabinoid receptor in pyramidal neurons of the hippocampus protects against seizure-induced excitotoxicity. PLoS One 2010; 5: e15707.

[85]   Das A, McDowell M, O'Dell CM *et al.* Post-treatment with voltage-gated Na(+) channel blocker attenuates kainic acid-induced apoptosis in rat primary hippocampal neurons. Neurochem Res 2010; 35: 2175-83.

[86]   Zeng LH, Rensing NR, Wong M. The mammalian target of rapamycin signaling pathway mediates epileptogenesis in a model of temporal lobe epilepsy. J Neurosci 2009; 29: 6964-72.

CHAPTER 8

Pilocarpine and Nerve Agents Induced Seizures: Similarities and Differences

Feng Ru Tang[1,3,*] and Weng Keong Loke[2]

[1]*Temasek Laboratories, National University of Singapore, 5A, Engineering Drive 1, Singapore 117411;* [2]*Defence Medical and Environmental Research Institute, DSO National Laboratories, 11 Stockport Road, Singapore 117605 and* [3]*Department of Anatomy, Yong Loo Lin School of Medicine, Block MD 10, National University of Singapore, 4 Medical Drive, Singapore 117597*

Abstract: Cholinergic nerve agents remain a realistic terrorist threat due to its combination of high lethality, demonstrated use and relative abundance of un-destroyed stockpiles around the world. While current fielded antidotes are able to mitigate acute poisoning, effective neuroprotection in the field remains a challenge amongst subjects with established status epilepticus (SE) following nerve agent intoxication. Due to ethical, safety and chemical security related issues, extensive preclinical and clinical research on cholinergic nerve agents is not possible. This may have been a contributory factor for the slow progress in uncovering uncovering new neuroprotectants for nerve agent casualties with established status epilepticus. To overcome this challenge, comparative research with surrogate chemicals that produce similar hypercholinergic toxicity but with less security concerns would be a useful approach forward. In this paper, we will systemically compare the mechanism of seizure generation, neuropathological, Genomic and neurobehavioral changes reported with pilocarpine, soman, and sarin challenged animal models. This review will be an important first step in closing this knowledge gap between two closely related models of neurotoxicity. Hopefully, it will spur further efforts in using surrogate cholinergic models by the wider scientific community to expedite the development of a new generation of antidotes that are better able to protect against delayed neurological effects inflicted by nerve agents.

INTRODUCTION

Recent studies have suggested that pilocarpine-induced status epilepticus (SE) model may be useful in studying the molecular mechanisms of neuropathology following exposure to chemical warfare nerve agents (CWNA) [1, 2]. Due to the similarities in physiological changes in the hippocampus [2], onset of seizure development, temperature effect and in the neuropathological changes in different regions of the brain between soman and pilocarpine models of seizure [1], the latter was proposed as a potential model to screen for neuroprotectants against nerve agents. Thus far, due to safety and surety related concerns, experimental studies on cholinergic nerve agents is largely limited to laboratories managed by or linked to military establishments. In contrast, the pilocarpine SE model is widely used in academia research and a wealth of research studies has been published on this model [3-23]. It remains unclear whether neuropathological mechanism findings from the pilocarpine SE model could be extrapolated directly to nerve agent-induced seizure effects.

In this paper, using data gathered from a wealth of reported studies in the last decade, we will systemically compare the mechanisms of seizure generation, subsequent neuropathological, genomic, and neurobehavioral changes reported with the pilocarpine-induced SE model against similar status epilepticus (SE) studies carried out with nerve agents (soman and sarin). This review will attempt to discern the key similarities and differences between the pilocarpine- and nerve agents-induced seizures, and discuss the feasibility of using the pilocarpine SE model as a surrogate research model to develop neuroprotectants against nerve agents.

CHEMISTRY, PHARMACOLOGY AND REPORTED APPLICATIONS OF PILOCARPINE, SOMAN AND SARIN

Pilocarpine

Pilocarpine is a naturally occurring imidazole alkaloid, first isolated in 1875 by Hardy and Gerrard from the leaves of Pilocarpus jaborandi [24] (Table **1**). It functions as a non-selective muscarinic receptor agonist and has been used to treat some types of glaucoma by increasing the outflow of fluid from the eye to reduce intra-ocular pressure [25]. Smaller doses are also used to induce salivation for collection of clinical samples for IgA antibody assay [26].

Address correspondence to Dr. Feng-Ru Tang: Temasek Laboratories, National University of Singapore, 5A Engineering Drive 1, #06-27, Singapore 117411. Tel: (65) 66011094; Fax: (65) 68726840; E-mail: tangfr@gmail.com

Pilocarpine is also reported to induce excessive sweating and salivation, bronchospasm, increased bronchial mucus secretion, tachycardia, hypertension, diarrhoea, brow-ache and miosis when used chronically as an eye drop. Accidental death arising from pilocarpine toxicity has been reported amongst hospital inpatients [27] and in victims with hypersensitivity to pilocarpine [28].

Systemic injection of pilocarpine can compromise the blood-brain barrier, which increased its penetration into the brain. Within the central nervous system, acting as a functional muscarinic agonist, it induces SE and temporal lobe epilepsy (TLE) in rodents. This property has been utilised as a means to study the physiology of TLE disorder and for investigating different treatment options for clinical TLE disorder [3, 6-8, 23, 29-32]. Pilocarpine has also been utilised as an antidote for scopolamine, atropine and hyoscyamine poisoning [33].

Soman (GD) and Sarin (GB)

Soman and sarin nerve agents are derivatives of phosphoric acids, with a fluorine leaving group linked directly to the phosphorus atom. Nerve agents disrupt the nervous system by inhibiting the synaptic cholinesterase enzyme. Inhibition occurs through the formation of a covalent bond between the phosphorus atom of nerve agents with the serine residue in acetycholinesterase catalytic site, resulting in the release of the fluoride anion as hydrogen fluoride. With the enzyme catalytic site inhibited, acetylcholine builds up in the synapse and continues to propagate post-synaptic nervous impulses, resulting in depolarisation block, hypersecretions, fasciculations, tremor, motor convulsions and respiratory distress (Table **1**).

Soman (GD), which has the chemical name pinacolyl methylphosphonofluoridate, was discovered in 1944 in Germany by Richard Kuhn. Soman is less volatile than Sarin and appears as a colorless liquid with a faint odour when pure. When impure, it has a yellow to brown color and a stronger odour described as camphor. Soman consists of a mixture of four stereoisomers, ranging from C(-) P (-), C(-) P(+), C(+) P (-) and C(+) P(+) [34]. Of the four, the C($\pm$)P(+) stereoisomers are at least 50 times less toxic compared to their C($\pm$)P(-) counterparts. Acetylcholinesterase inhibited by C(-)P(-)-soman was also harder to reactivate with oximes as compared with those inhibited by C(+)P(-)-soman.

Sarin (GB), which has the chemical name methylphosphonofluoridic acid, (1-methylethyl) ester, was discovered in 1938 in Wuppertal-Elberfeld, Germany during efforts to create more potent pesticides. Sarin, the most volatile of four nerve agents made during the 2nd World War, is synthesized by reacting isopropanol and methylphosphonic acid difluoride [35]. Sarin has two main stereoisomers, P(+)- sarin and P(-)-sarin, the latter being more toxic of the 2 isomers [34]. With modern binary technology, Sarin could be formed in-situ by mixing these two separate, relatively non-toxic compounds - (a) methylphosphonyl difluoride and (b) a mixture of isopropyl alcohol and isopropyl amine, immediately after firing the weapon. Sarin is rapidly hydrolyzed in acidic, neutral and basic media producing different products.

Unlike pilocarpine, sarin and soman are developed solely as potential military offensive weapons. Sarin has been used by Iraq against Iranian forces during the Iran-Iraq War (1983-1988) and again by Iraqi forces on their own Kurdish population in 1988. It was employed by Aum Shinrikyo sect in two terrorist attacks in Japan in 1994 (Matsumoto, Nagano, 7 fatalities) and subsequently in 1995 (Tokyo Subway, 12 fatalities). Unlike pilocarpine, there has been no reported clinical applications for nerve agents and all existing research are restricted to uncovering their toxic effects and development of medical countermeasures against such toxic effects.

MECHANISM OF SEIZURE GENERATION FOLLOWING PILOCARPINE, SOMAN AND SARIN CHALLENGE

Pilocarpine

During the early stages of pilocarpine-induced status epilepticus (PISE), cholinergic elements play a predominant role in seizures initiation and propagation as seizure events could be blocked by atropine or attenuated by hemicholinium-3. The latter being a potent inhibitor of high-affinity choline transporter, leads to inhibition of acetylcholine synthesis and availability for synaptic release, thereby attenuating cholinergic transmission. Once status epilepticus is established, atropine administration alone could no longer control seizures, suggesting that non-cholinergic elements such as glutamate, GABA and dopamine are involved in the maintenance of seizures [36-38]. This deduction is supported by the observed anti-convulsive effects displayed by antagonist compounds to NMDA

[39] and kainate [40] receptors, by stimulation of striatal dopamine D2 receptors [41] or by a substantial loss of glutamic acid decarboxylase (GAD) mRNA-containing neurons [42].

However, recent studies have revealed that postsynaptic adenosine A(1) and A(2a) receptors may also be involved in seizure generation as activation of A(1) receptor by agonist 2-chloroadenosine (2-CADO) or blocking A(2a) receptor by antagonist SCH 58261 could reduce seizure activity [43]. On the other hand, findings from our group have revealed that targeting metabotropic glutamate receptors (mGluRs), in particular mGluR5, may be able to control pilocarpine-induced seizures and subsequent neuronal damage [13]. Furthermore, we have also observed significant changes in expression of chemokine receptors such as CCR7, CCR8, CCR9 and CCR10 [17], CCR3, CCR2A, levels of macrophage inflammatory protein 1-alpha (MIP-1alpha), monocyte chemotactic protein-1 (MCP-1) [21], calcium channels such as Ca(v)1.2, Ca(v)1.3 (L-type), Ca(v)2.1 (P/Q-type), and Cav2.2 [20, 22] within the mouse hippocampus during acute stages of PISE.

Combined with a recent report that intravenous administration of IL-1 receptor antagonist (IL-1ra) may prevent pilocarpine-induced seizures and blood-brain barrier (BBB) damage, or administration of calcium channel blocker, nimodipine, inhibited convulsions, SE and significantly lowered mortality and cerebral changes [44], it challenges prior suggestions that pilocarpine-induced seizures are initiated and maintained solely by neurotransmitters and their receptors. Instead, it seems that calcium channels, cytokines, chemokines and their receptors may also play a pivotal role in pilocarpine induced status epilepticus.

Soman

Three phases of seizure development were reported in the development of status epilepticus during Soman intoxication, namely (a) an early cholinergic phase (pre-seizure to ca. 5 min after seizure onset), (b) a transitional phase (> 5 to < 40 min) of progressively mixed cholinergic/non-cholinergic modulation, and finally, (c) a non-cholinergic phase (> 40 min) maintaining status epilepticus [45]. The onset and earliest phase of nerve agent-induced seizures was reported to be controlled almost exclusively by cholinergic mechanisms.

During the transition phase, between 5 and 40 min of on-going seizures, there appeared to be diminishing cholinergic control over the seizure activities. Significant decreases in norepinephrine (NE) content were reported along with significant increases in dopamine (DA) and DA metabolites such as 3,4-dihydroxyphenylacetic acid (DOPAC) and homovanillic acid (HVA). During this period, glutamate release was reported to increase significantly in limbic regions of the brain [46-47]. Thus, during this transition phase, there appears to be increasing involvement of other neurotransmitter systems recruited by the seizure process with diminishing cholinergic control per se over the seizure activity.

Forty minutes after seizure development, the cholinergic system appears to have minimal control over on-going status epilepticus as non-cholinergic processes, in particular excitatory amino acid (EAA) processes appears to facilitate SE, as suggested by successful seizures termination using antagonists of NMDA or AMPA or kainate receptors [45-49].

Besides cholinergic and glutamate neurotransmitter systems, dopaminergic neurotransmission was also reported to have a role in mediating nerve agent induced neurotoxicity as D1-like receptor antagonist (SCH 23390, halobenzazepine(R)-(+)-7-chloro-8-hydroxy -3-methyl-1-phenyl-2,3,4,5 -tetrahydro-1H-3-benzazepine) was reported to prevent clinical signs associated with Soman poisoning [50-51], possibly through activation of the striatonigral GABAergic pathway [52]. In addition, Bodjarian *et al.* (1995) demonstrated that histamine H1 subtypes and mGluRs contributed to increase in inositol 1,4,5-triphosphate (IP3) during early seizures, which suggested that these alternate receptors might also be involved in the initiation and maintenance of Soman-induced seizures [53].

Sarin

Sarin-induced seizures could be effectively controlled at early stages by atropine in the rat and guinea pig models, suggesting again the involvement of cholinergic elements in seizures initiation [54]. Application of the adenosine A(1) receptor agonist N(6)-cyclopentyladenosine (CPA) or the partial adenosine A(1) receptor agonists 2-deoxy-N(6)-cyclopentyladenosine (2-deoxy-CPA) and 8-butylamino-N(6)-cyclopentyl- adenosine (8-butylamino-CPA) has been reported to abolish epileptiform activity in a concentration-related manner in Sarin-induced seizures, which suggests that adenosine A(1) receptor activation is involved in seizure initiation [55- 56].

When mapping the neural areas (lateral ventricle, anterior piriform cortex, basolateral amygdala, area tempestas) for the ability of three classes of drugs - muscarinic antagonists (scopolamine), benzodiazepines, and N-methyl-D-aspartate antagonists (MK-801), to moderate nerve agent induced seizure activities, Skovira [57] observe that scopolamine provides anticonvulsant effects in all areas tested, while midazolam is effective in all areas except the lateral ventricle. On the other hand, MK-801 is only effective at preventing seizures when micro-injected directly into the basolateral amygdala or area tempestas of the rat brain. This finding suggests the existence of unique neuroanatomical and pharmacological specificity for control of nerve agent-induced seizures. The demonstration of central neuro-inflammatory processes following Sarin exposure suggests that cytokine receptors are also involved in seizures maintenance and the consequent long-term brain damage arising from seizures [58].

NEUROPATHOLOGY OBSERVED POST PILOCARPINE, SOMAN AND SARIN CHALLENGE

Neuronal Damage

Pilocarpine

In the pilocarpine model, status epilepticus induces neuronal damage in many different brain regions such as the olfactory cortex, amygdaloid complex, thalamus, hippocampus, subiculum, piriform and entorhinal cortices, neocortex, and substantia nigra [3-12, 14-16, 23]. The patterns of neuronal loss reported vary among animal species, strains and within the same animal strain. Different patterns are also reported among many research groups.

In the mouse hippocampus, a significant loss of hilar neurons in the dentate gyrus has been reported as early as 1 day after PISE. However, loss of pyramidal neurons in CA1-3 areas was not obvious at acute stages during and immediately after PISE. However, by 7 and 60 days after PISE, most neurons in the stratum pyramidale of CA1 and CA3 areas and in the hilus of the dentate gyrus are reported to have disappeared. The number of interneurons marked by calcium-binding proteins such as calbindin (CB), calretinin (CR) and parvalbumin (PV) in CA1-3 areas is also reported to have decreased [12]. Mossy cells in the hilus of the dentate gyrus labeled by glutamate receptor 1 (GluR1) or CR disappear almost completely [11-12, 14, 59].

In the lateral entorhinal cortex (LEnt), there is a significant loss of total neurons in layers II-VI in experimental mice at 2 months after PISE [15, 59]. Loss of CB (51%), CR (49%) and PV (44%) immunopositive neurons becomes very obvious. Furthermore, drastic loss of CR-immunopositive axonal plexuses is reported in layers V-VI [15, 60].

In the dorsal subiculum (Dsub), 15% of neurons are lost at 2 months after PISE [23]. Loss of PV (34%), CB (47%) and CR (19%) immunopositive interneurons is also much more significant than the loss of total neurons stained with NeuN immunocytochemistry [23].

Neuronal loss in the lateral, basal, and accessory basal nuclei of the amygdale is about 34.4%, 28.7% and 43.1% respectively at 2 months after PISE. Of the three subtypes of CB, CR and PV-immunopositive interneurons in the lateral, basal or accessory basal nucleus, 33.5%, 13.5%, or 26.4% of CB, 48.1%, 36.9% or 36.4% of CR, 29.9%, 35.1% or 15.5% of PV-immunopositive neurons disappear in each nucleus respectively (Tang *et al.*, unpublished data).

Soman

It has been well documented that a single dose of soman induces acute brain pathology in laboratory animals [61-65]. In Nauta and the Fink-Heimer staining (*i.e.*, the techniques used for degenerated axons and their terminals) of brain sections from rats challenged with soman, axon degeneration is observed in the cerebral cortex, basal ganglia, thalamus, subthalamic region, hypothalamus, hippocampus, fornix, septum, preoptic area, superior colliculus, pretectal area, basilar pontine nuclei, medullary tegmentum and corticospinal tracts [61].

Pathological study shows that at 1 or 6 hrs after injection of 140, 120, or 100µg/kg of soman, only diffuse congestion is observed. However, twenty four hours after poisoning, neuronal degeneration is reported in many brain regions including piriform cortex (layer II), locus coeruleus, piriform cortex (layer III), entorhinal cortex, endopiriform nucleus, olfactory tublercle, anterior olfactory nucleus, olfactory bulb, cerebral cortex, thalamus, caudate-putamen, dentate gyrus, hippocampus, inferior colliculus, accumbent nucleus, copus geniculatum, lateral ventricle, amygdale, lateral septal nucleus, thalamus, subiculum, neocortex, claustrum, cerebellum, globus pallidus, frontal cortex, substantia nigra [62-66].

McDonough *et al.* (1998) report observations of sustained damage in all cortical areas, with piriform and perirhinal cortices exhibiting the most severe pathological change. Subcortical limbic areas (amygdala, amygdala-piriform transition zone, hippocampus, claustrum) and various thalamic nuclei are consistently the most severely damaged brain regions in all animals regardless of survival time. Brainstem structures, cerebellum, spinal cord, and other motor output nuclei are, however, never damaged [67]. The severity of neuronal damage does not appear to be related to the doses of soman injected as long as status epilepticus is initiated.

The brain lesions in primates challenged by soman are limited to the hippocampus, amygdala, and thalamus (of one animal), and consisted of neuron necrosis and dropout, spongiosis, gliosis, astrocytosis, and vascularization [68]. Further study reveals a tight relationship between seizures activity and neuropathology in soman poisoning, which suggests that refined, standardized analysis of electrographic parameters drawn from electrocorticography (ECoG) tracings and power spectrum may serve as a useful tool to predict the presence, localization, and severity of soman-induced brain damage [69].

Sarin

Sarin induces brain damage in varying degrees of severity in about 70% of challenged animals, observed mainly in the hippocampus, piriform cortex, cerebellum and thalamus. The damage is exacerbated with time and at three months post exposure, it extends to regions which were initially not affected. Morphometric analysis reveals a significant decline in the number of CA1 hippocampal cells and reduction in CA1 and CA3 areas of the hippocampus. The neuropathological findings, although generally similar to those described following soman, differ in some features, unique to each compound, for example, frontal cortex damage is specific to soman poisoning [47, 58, 70-72].

Neurogenesis

In the pilocarpine model, dentate granule cell neurogenesis has been reported to increase at early stages, but decrease at chronic stages after pilocarpine injection [11-12, 73-76]. Parent *et al.* (1997) indicated that seizure activity induces a marked increase in dentate granule cell neurogenesis at 3, 6, and 13 days but not at 27 days or 1 year after PISE [73]. Newly differentiated dentate granule cells are integrated into abnormal hippocampal network, which may play an important role in epileptogenesis [75]. Varodayan *et al.* (2009) observed increased cell proliferation in the dentate gyrus commencing at 2 hrs post-SE, which is sustained for a further 40 days, suggesting that a "decrease in cell-cycle length of dentate gyrus progenitors is at least partially responsible for increased numbers of newborn cells following SE" [77].

Jung et al. (2009) showed that the majority of newly generated cells in the extrahippocampal areas proliferate in-situ, and differentiate mainly into astrocytes or oligodendrocytes. In addition, stromal cell-derived factor-1-alpha is found to be induced in close temporal and anatomical association with seizure-induced plasticity [78]. In our own studies, we also consistently observe drastic reduction in neuronal number in the sub-granular layer of the dentate gyrus at the chronic stage after PISE [11-12]. These findings are in agreement with previous studies obtained from the kainic acid model [79-81]. Based on their elegant studies [79], Hattiangady and Shetty (2009) concluded that "severely diminished dentate gyrus (DG) neurogenesis in TLE was not associated with either decreased production of new cells or with reduced survival of newly born cells in the sub-granular zone-granule cell layer (SGZ-GCL). Rather, it was linked to a dramatic decline in the neuronal fate-choice decision of newly generated cells". In another words, "the differentiation of newly born cells changed mainly into glia cells with chronic TLE from predominantly neuronal differentiation seen in control conditions" [81]. The same principle may also be applied to the mouse pilocarpine model as few NeuroD and doublecortin (DCX) immunpositive neurons could be found in the subgranlar layer of the dentate gyrus. Moreover, astrocytic gliosis is very obvious in the hippocampus at chronic stages after SE.

In comparison, at early stages post-soman poisoning (3 and 8 days post-soman poisoning), neural progenitor proliferation increases significantly in the subgranular zone of the dentate gyrus (SGZ) and the subventricular zone (SVZ). This increased proliferation rate is detected up to 1 month post-soman poisoning [82]. However, generation of new neurons in the subgranular layer of the dentate gyrus was actually reduced post-soman poisoning. Interestingly, viable neural progenitors were located in the SGZ or in the SVZ of the brain post soman poisoning. Similar observations were also made by other research groups [83, 84].

In the amygdala of mice, delayed neuronal regeneration occurs between 60 and 90 days post-soman poisoning [82]. A massive short-termed microgliosis peaks at day 3 post-soman poisoning whereas delayed astrogliosis is observed from 3 to 90 days after soman poisoning. On the other hand, oligodendroglial cells or their precursors are reported to be almost unaffected by soman poisoning [82].

Axonal and Dendritic Architectonic Changes

In the hippocampus of the mouse pilocarpine model, sprouted mossy fibers are consistently detected in the inner molecular layer of the dentate gyrus using both Timm staining [29] and phaseolus vulgaris leucoagglutinin (PHA-L) anterograde tracing techniques [11]. Sprouted mossy fibers with PHA-L immunopositive staining are also observed to extend to as far as the CA1 area to establish synaptic connections with glutamate receptor 1 [11], calbindin, calretinin and parvalbumin [16] immunpositive neurons in the CA1 area. When PHA-L is injected into CA3 area, sprouted Schaffer collaterals with increased number of larger boutons are demonstrated to establish perisomatic contact with neurons in the stratum pyramidale in CA1 area of the hippocampus in SE mice [14].

Further study indicates that sprouted PHA-L immunopositive axon terminals and boutons made contact with CB-, CR-, and PV- immunopositive neurons, which suggested the existence of forward inhibition in the CA1 area mediated from the CA3 area [14]. In the hippocampus of experimental mice, newly sprouted dendrites with cone-like dendritic spines were also shown in the CA1 and CA3 areas. These dendrites and dendritic spines are glutamate receptor 1 immunopositive [11-12]. In the afferent pathways from the entorhinal cortex, the enlarged PHA-L immunopositive en passant and terminal boutons aggregate to form clusters of grape-like structures in different parts of the dentate gyrus. which included the hilus, molecular layer and stratum granulosum, of experimental mice at 1 year after PISE [15].

In the subiculum, the density of dendritic spines in the 2nd and 3rd order dendrites of pyramidal neurons is significantly higher in pilocarpine-treated mice at 2 months after SE. However, in the interneurons, the density of dendritic spines in the 3rd and 4th order dendrites was significantly reduced when compared to control animals [23]. Sprouted axons with en passant and terminal boutons from neurons in the entorhinal cortex were also reported in the subiculum, amygdale and perirhinal cortex at 2 months and one year after SE. However, there was a significant reduction of contacts between choline acetyltransferase (ChAT) immunopositive neurons and PHA-L labeled en passant and terminal boutons in the striatum.

In the afferent pathways of the lateral entorhinal cortex (LEnt), significant reductions in projections from the piriform cortex/endopiriform, amygdale and reunions thalamic nucleus to LEnt are observed in mice 1 year after PISE [15]. In the efferent pathway of the basolateral amygdale (BLA) in the mouse pilocarpine model, sprouted axons and enlarged PHA-L immunopositive en passant and terminal boutons are demonstrated in the ventral subiculum (vSub) and the perirhinal cortex (PRh), particularly in the latter. Some of these axon en passant and terminal boutons are extremely large. In the afferent, much fewer neurons in vSub and the layer V of LEnt are demonstrated to project to the BLA (Tang *et al.*, unpublished data).

In the soman model, mossy fiber sprouting has been reported in CA2 area of the hippocampus at 3 months after soman intoxication [83]. However, in sarin-treated animal, axon sprouting is found in the peripheral nervous system, where axonal degeneration is accompanied by junctional and extrajunctional membrane depolarization, which is followed by nerve sprouting at focal, distal, and terminal nerve fibers [85]. New ectopic endings, originating from the same endplate, were discovered adjacent to the terminal axon and also distant from the parent endplate. Very elaborate terminal arborization and occasional multi-branching arose from a progressive growth sprout. The new sprouting may play a role in compensating for the loss of synaptic contact caused by sarin [85].

GENOMIC RESPONSES DURING AND AFTER PILOCARPINE-, SOMAN-AND SARIN-INDUCED SEIZURES

Pilocarine

Genomic responses to PISE comprise of distinct patterns at different stages of epileptogenesis. At day 3 after PISE, immediate early/stress-related genes and genes for growth and differentiation, such as insulin growth factor-binding protein and heparin binding epidermal growth factor-like growth factor, are reported to be up-regulated in CA1 area and dentate gyrus. Genes involved in transcriptional regulation, such as VGF-inducible nerve growth factor and thyroid hormone receptor, were also up-regulated in the dentate gyrus. Induction of genes for cellular reorganization and reactivation of developmental programmes, such as cdc2a, and for structural remodeling, such as tenascin-C, are also observed while mitogen activated protein 2 (MAP2) transcript, is reduced. However, mitogen-activated protein kinase kinase kinase 1 (MEKK1), a molecule known to promote neuronal apoptosis, is selectively up-regulated in the CA1 area.

At day 14 after PISE, induction of genes involved in second messenger signaling, transcriptional regulation, cellular and structural reorganization, neuronal cytoskeleton-plasma membrane interactions, growth cone formation, cellular reorganization, hippocampal remodeling, synaptic reorganization, and tubulogenesis was observed. At the chronic epileptic stage, substantial increase of gene transcripts for neurotransmitter receptors and ion channels, was also observed [86]. Overall, it appeared that 14 days after PISE, a much higher percentage of the genes up-regulated were involved in either injury response or cell survival, whereas a modest predominance of metabolic, morphology and extracellular signaling genes were amongst those down-regulated [87].

Soman

Soman challenge induced modulation of a wide variety of biological functions in animals as revealed by gene ontology mapping of the hippocampus [88]. One hour post-exposure, neurotrophin/tyrosine kinase receptor (TRK), p38 mitogen activated protein kinase (MAPK), extracellular signal-regulated kinase (ERK)/MAPK, cyclic adenosine-3', 5'-monophosphate (cAMP), and interleukin-6 (IL-6) signaling were the most significantly modulated pathways. At 3 hours, genes regulating peroxisome-proliferator activated receptor (PPAR), IL-10, IL-6, neurotrophin/TRK, and Toll-like receptor signaling were also significantly modulated. The most significantly modulated canonical pathways at 6 hours post-exposure included neurotrophin/TRK signaling, valine leucine and isoleucine biosynthesis, IL-6, G-protein coupled receptor signaling, cAMP-mediated signaling, IL-10, epidermal growth factor (EGF), and PPAR signaling. At 12 hours post-exposure, IL-10, IL-6, acute phase response, p38 MAPK, death receptor, Toll-like receptor, nuclear factor-κα B (NF-κB), PPAR and neurotrophin/ TRK signaling were among the most significantly modulated canonical pathways.

Glucocorticoid receptor, insulin-like growth factor (IGF-1), p53, PPAR, IL-6 signaling, aminoacyl-tRNA biosynthesis, and EGF signaling were the more significantly modulated canonical pathways at 1 day post-exposure. At 2 days post-exposure, coagulation system, IL-10, acute phase response and IL-6 signaling, GM-CSF, glutamate, glycerophospholipid, arginine, proline and glycerolipid metabolism, phospholipid degradation, are the most significantly modulated canonical pathways. At 3 days, the most significantly modulated canonical pathways are the complement system, ephrin receptor, acute phase response, apoptosis, integrin and IL-10 signaling, N-glycanand phospholipid degradation as well as, glycosaminoglycan and glycerophospholipid metabolism.

Four days following soman poisoning, the complement system, acute phase response, ephrin receptor, granulocyte-macrophage colony stimulating factor (GM-CSF), extracellular signal-regulated kinases/ mitogen-activated protein kinases (ERK/MAPK), interferon, IL-6 signaling, antigen presentation pathway and the one carbon pool by folate pathway were among the most significantly changed pathways.

At 1 week, p38 MAPK signaling, glutamate metabolism, acute phase response signaling, alanine and aspartate metabolism, interferon signaling, hepatic fibrosis/hepatic stellate cell activation, complement system, fibroblast growth factor (FGF) signaling, and metabolism of D-glutamine and D-glutamate were the most significantly modulated canonical pathways [88]. In summary, soman poisoning appears to induce genes regulating numerous signaling and inflammatory pathways.

Sarin

Microarray analysis indicated significant changes in gene expression profiles at an early time point (15 min) after sarin challenge. These genes fall into the following categories: 1) cytoskeletal and cell adhesion molecules, 2) ion channels, 3) neuropeptide and their receptors, 4) calcium channels and binding proteins, 5) chemokines and their receptors, 6) G-protein coupled receptor and related molecules, 7) purigenic signaling molecules, 8) cholinergic signaling, 9) energy metabolism, 10) GABAnergic signaling, 11) glutamatergic and aspartate signaling, 12) mitochondria associated proteins, 13) myelin proteins, 14) neurotransmission and related transporters, 15) serotonergic signaling, 16) tyrosine phosphorylation molecules, 17) ATPases and ATP-based transporters, 18) catecholaminergic signaling, 19) cyclic nucleotide signaling, 20) cytokines and their receptors, 21) nitric oxide signaling, 22) tumor necrosis factor (TNF) beta family, 23) transcription factors [89].

At 2 hrs, more genes for ion (8 genes) and calcium channel as well as binding proteins (6 genes) were altered than those for other groups such as ATPases and ATP-based transporters, growth factors, G-protein-coupled receptor pathway-related molecules, neurotransmission and neurotransmitter transporters, cytoskeletal and cell adhesion molecules, hormones, mitochondria-associated proteins, myelin proteins, stress-activated molecules, cytokine, caspase, GABAnergic, glutamatergic, immediate early gene, prostaglandin, transcription factor, and tyrosine phosphorylation molecule. Persistent alteration of the following genes was also noted: beta-arrestin 1 (Arrb1), Ca2+/calmodulin-dependent protein kinases (CaMKIIa, CaMKIId), H(+)/Cl(-) exchange transporter 5 (Clcn5), IL-10, c-Kit (CD117) and proteolipid protein 1 (Plp1), suggesting altered G protein-coupled receptor (GPCR), kinase, channel, and cytokine pathways. Some of those genes such as glial fibrillary acidic protein (GFAP), Neurofilament High molecular weight protein (NF-H), CaMKIIa, Calmodulin (Calm), and myelin basic protein (MBP) are involved in the pathogenesis of sarin-induced pathology and suspected organophosphate-induced delayed neurotoxicity (OPIDN). Induction of both proapoptotic (Bcl2l11, Casp6) and antiapoptotic (Bcl-X) genes, besides suppression of p21, suggests complex cell death/protection-related mechanisms were operating during early stages of sarin induced SE.

Principal component analysis (PCA) of the expression data confirms that the changes in gene expression are a function of sarin exposure since the control and treatment groups response are clearly distinguished. Following sarin poisoning, both degenerative and regenerative pathways are activated early and contributed to the level of neurodegeneration and neuropathological alterations observed at a later time [90]. At chronic stages (3 months) following sarin challenge, the number of altered genes was highest for calcium channels and binding proteins, as well as for immediate early genes [89]. Genes for cytoskeletal and cell adhesion molecules, GABAnergic signaling, growth factors and inhibitors, cyclic nucleotide signaling, cytokines and their receptors, ion channels, synaptic vesicle proteins and transporters, catecholamine signaling, chemokines, death factors, G-protein coupled receptors, glutamatergic and aspartate signaling, metabolism, proteases, Rho family of guanosine triphosphatases (Rho-GTPase) effector and tyrosine kinases, have also changed. Those for cyclic nucleotide signaling, cytokines and their receptors, G-protein coupled receptor, glutamate receptor all α-amino-3-hydroxy-5-methyl-4-isoxazolepropionic acid (AMPA) subtype, growth factors and inhibitors, metabolism, and proteases, were up-regulated. On the other hand, genes for catecholaminergic, chemokine and their receptors, death factors, immediate early genes, Rho-GTPase effector, transporters, and tyrosine kinases were down-regulated [89].

LONG-TERM EFFECTS OF PILOCARPINE, SOMAN AND SARIN ON BEHAVIOURAL RESPONSE

Pilocarpine

Learning and memory impairment in pilocarpine model has been detected not only in adult rats [91-96], but also in immature ones as early as at postnatal days 7, 8, 9 [95-101]. The impairment could be improved by voluntary physical activity and environmental enrichment [96, 98, 102]. However, antiepileptic drugs such as carbamazepine [92] and levetiracetam [94] do not alleviate compromised visual-spatial memory performances of PISE animals in the Morris water-maze. In pilocarpine model, depression [93, 103-106] or anxiety [93, 95] was reported. Recent studies indicated that depression could be improved by treatment with human recombinant Interleukin-1 receptor antagonist (IL-1ra) [104] or Bacopa monnieri extract through the 5-HT (2C) receptor [106].

Soman

Soman (at doses less than or equal to 3% LD50) interferes with two-way shuttlebox avoidance learning, open field behavior, and complex coordinated movements (hurdle -stepping task). These findings suggested that paradigms that involved higher central nervous system (CNS) structures and required motor activity are sensitive to cholinesterase (ChE) inhibitors at doses far lower than those that cause overt symptoms [107]. Soman also induced anxiety-like behavior profile when animals were tested 30 days after intoxication [108]. The decrement in learning ability was observed in both soman-poisoned controls and those that received oxime/atropine-treatment [84]. It thus appears that a therapeutic regime involving oximes-reactivation of organophosphate-inhibited enzyme, anticholinergic treatment with atropine and administration of the anti-epileptic drug diazepam did not provide complete protection of the CNS and long-term neuronal deficits will still be observed amongst animals surviving lethal soman poisoning [83, 109-112].

Sarin

Sarin at a dosage of 71 mg/kg (43% LD50) induced conditioned flavor aversion. When compared to vehicle controls, the animals' spontaneous locomotor activities were increased when sarin was given at 61 mg/kg (37% LD50), but decreased significantly when dosages were raised to 84 mg/kg (51% LD50) and 115 mg/kg (70% LD50). Significant decrement in rotorod performance was observed at 98 and 115 mg/kg (sarin LD50 reported as 165 mg/kg) [107, 113].

In sarin poisoned rats, Grauer *et al.* (2008) observed significant increases in overall activity with no habituation over days in the open field test at six weeks, four and six months after sarin exposure. In a working memory paradigm water maze test, these same rats show impaired working and reference memory processes with no recovery [72]. It is consistent with other studies showing that inhalation exposure to sarin at levels even below those causing overt signs of clinical toxicity could produce cognitive and performance deficits [114-117]. Sub-toxic exposures to sarin also produce neurodevelopmental deficits [118]. Moreover, repeated sarin exposure may disrupt normal sleeping patterns (*i.e.*, lower frequency bandwidths) [119].

In human, symptomatic sequelae to sarin exposure are observed in the higher and visual nervous system 6–8 months after sarin exposure amongst Tokyo rail commuters [120]. Delayed effects on psychomotor performance following the sarin poisoning are also reported [121-122]. Rescue workers and police officers suffer a chronic decline of memory function 3 years after the sarin poisoning in Tokyo [123]. Similar symptoms were reported amongst other casualties of sarin terror attacks in Japan [124].

Hence, it appears that at acutely non-toxic doses, both sarin and soman affect the behavior of rats but the behavioural reaction profiles of animals treated with these 2 nerve agents differ from each other [125]. While both soman and sarin affected the behavior of rats in the plus-maze test and have inactivating effects on the behavior of rats [126], only sarin impaired motor coordination/balance. Furthermore, sarin could also enhance acoustic startle, decrease distance explored in the open field [127], cause sensorimotor impairments [128] and post-traumatic stress disorder [129-131].

SUMMARY

Extensive studies have been undertaken with pilocarpine-induced seizures, which correlated with its easy availability since it is not a chemical under surety control. Animals with PISE developed epilepsy that imitates many characteristics of patients with TLE [132-133]. Ability to use the pilocarpine model as a surrogate nerve agent SE model may help in efforts to uncover new drug targets that could control the acute and subsequent neurological and neuropsychological diseases arising from SE in all 3 models.

Comparison with data from current research on soman and sarin (refer to Table **I**) suggests that there are many key similarities between pilocarpine- and soman- or sarin-induced seizures that includes : 1) seizure is initiated by cholinergic elements and maintained by non-cholinergic ones, 2) there is high mortality within 24hrs of intoxication [2, 54], 3) neuropathological changes occurred in the hippocampus, pyriform and entorhinal cortices, amygdale, thalamus, *etc.*, at chronic stages after SE, 4) similar neurobehavioral changes such as learning memory impairment, anxiety, depression etc are observed in both pilocarpine and nerve agent challenged animals, 5) at early stages after intoxication, atropine could effectively control the cholinergic crisis induced by these 3 agents.

However, when analyzing glucose cortical utilization (CGU) in four cerebral cortex and thirty-five subcortical regions in pyridostigmine-soman and Li-pilocarpine models of cholinergic seizures, Scremin *et al.* (1998) reported significantly different patterns obtained with each model, *i.e.*, pyridostigmine-soman treatment activated CGU in all structures with the exception of the inferior colliculus. On the other hand, Li-pilocarpine treatment increased CGU in all forebrain structures with the exception of habenula and diagonal band. Moreover, no activation was demonstrated in the brainstem (except substantia nigra), while inhibition of CGU was observed in the inferior colliculus. In contrast, Li-physostigmine induced profound CGU inhibition in all areas of cerebral cortex while activating globus pallidus, entopenduncular nucleus, and substantia nigra [134].

Henceforth, additional studies with nerve agent models in the following areas will be needed to clarify some important issues relevant to each model to enable a more definitive conclusion on the applicability of the pilocarpine model as a surrogate model to study nerve agent induced SE effects:

1. Long-term video and electroencephalography (EEG) monitoring in sarin or soman model may be useful to clarify whether animals challenged with nerve agents develop epilepsy after SE as

commonly reported with pilocarpine model. Uncovering such effects will also lead to development of new therapeutic strategies to prevent epileptogenesis in casualties of nerve agent intoxication.

2. Systemic study of neurogenesis, axon reorganization and growth of dendritic spines in limbic system of the animal model of sarin or soman may provide evidence to explain how and why neurological and neuropsychological diseases are developed after nerve agent poisoning. This would allow one to develop new strategies to prevent the occurrence of those pathological changes and the subsequent diseases.

3. Detailed investigation of neuropathological changes and related molecular biological mechanism in sarin or soman model may provide evidence to elucidate different mechanisms of pathophysiological changes in each model. This will help to develop new generation antidotes with both anticonvulsive and neuroprotective effects at early stages after intoxication. The new generation antidotes could have common targets on pathological conditions appearing post intoxication by different nerve agents, or may be specific to those caused by one particular nerve agent.

4. Comparable parameters such as time points after intoxication, gene categorization and animal strains may need to be standardised for investigations on genomic, proteomic and lipidomic responses after soman or sarin challenge so as to permit comparison with changes in the pilocarpine model. This is because data gathered from existing studies, which have not standardized such factors, may be affected by those factors, which therefore do not permit conclusive comparisons.

Table 1: Similarities and differences after pilocarpine-, soman- and sarin-induced seizures

	Pilocarpine $(C_{11}H_{16}N_2O_2)$	Sarin $(C_4H_{10}FO_2P)$	Soman $(C_7H_{16}FO_2P)$	Similarities	Differences
Structures				No similarty between pilocarpine and nerve agents	Pilocarpine is an imidazole alkaloid, whereas sarin and soman are organophosphates
Targets	Muscarinic receptor (agonists)	Cholinesterase (ChE) (inhibitor)	ChE (inhibitor)	All of them target on cholinergic system. Soman and sarin have the same target	Pilocarpine is acting on muscarinic receptor, sarin and soman on cholinesterase
Mechanism of seizure generation	1) Initiation of seizure by activation of muscarinic receptor 2) Maintenance of seizures by glutamate, GABA, dopamine 3) Other molecules such as adenosine receptors, cytokines, chemokines and their receptors, calcium channels etc, may also be involved in maintenance of status epilepticus and onset of spontaneously recurrent seizures	Initiation of seizure by cholinergic elements, Histamine H1 subtypes and metabotropic glutamate receptors Maintenance of seizures by mixed cholinergic/ non-cholinergic (including glutamate, GABA, dopamine) modulation	1) Initiation of seizure by cholinergic elements and adenosine A(1) receptor activation. 2) Non-cholinergic elements (including glutamate, GABA, dopamine) in unique neuroanatomical location, and cytokine receptors are also involved in seizure generation	Seizure is initiated by cholinergic elements and maintained by glutamate, GABA, dopamine systems	Histamine H1 subtypes and metabotropic glutamate receptors are involved in the initiation of sarin induced seizure, whereas adenosine A(1) receptor may initiate soman-induced seizure. Calcium channels, chemokines and their receptors may be involved in maintenance of pilocarpine induced seizure, and in onset of epilepsy

Pathology	**Axons and dendrites**	Axon sprouting and newly sprouted dendrites with growth cone-like dendritic spines are found in the limbic system at chronic stages after PISE 4)	Axon sprouting occurs in the peripheral nervous system	Mossy fiber sprouting is observed in CA2 area of the hippocampus at 3 months after soman intoxication	No similarty between pilocarpine- and nerve agents- induced axon sprouting	Mossy fiber sprouting is observed in CA2 area of the hippocampus after soman intoxication, but in CA3 area after pilocarpine treatment
	Neuron damage	Loss of neurons, in particular, interneurons occurs in the hippocampus, amygdaloid complex, thalamus, subiculum, piriform and entorhinal cortices, neocortex, and substantia nigra	Neuronal loss reported to occur mainly in the hippocampus, piriform cortex, amygdala cerebellum and thalamus	Loss of neurons reported in piriform cortex, locus coeruleus, entorhinal cortex, endopiriform nucleus, olfactory tublercle, anterior olfactory nucleus, olfactory bulb, cerebral cortex, thalamus, caudate-putamen, dentate gyrus, hippocampus, inferior colliculus, accumbent nucleus, corpus geniculatum, lateral ventricle, amygdale, lateral septal nucleus, thalamus, subiculum, neocortex, claustrum, cerebellum, globus pallidus, frontal cortex, substantia nigra	Hippocampus, piriform cortex, amygdale, thalamus	Nerve agents induce neuronal loss in cerebellum. Soman induces neuronal loss in the frontal cortex, but sarin does not produce similar damage. Pilocarpine does not induce neuronal damage in the cerebellum and frontal cortex
	Neurogenesis	The dentate granule cell neurogenesis is increased at early stages (first 3 weeks) after pilocarpine induced status epilepticus (PISE), but decreased thereafter	No report	There is a transient decrease of neural progenitor proliferation on day 1 post-exposure in the subgranular zone. Elevated neural precursor replication occurs from post-soman days 3 to 30, with a peak on post-soman day 8. By 90 days after soman challenging, neural progenitor proliferation is significantly reduced	Neurogenesis increases in the subgranular zone from day 3 until 3 weeks after intoxication with pilocarpine or soman, and decreases thereafter.	There is a transient decrease of neural progenitor proliferation on day 1 post-soman exposure in the subgranular zone

	Up-regulated genes	Up-regulated genes	Up-regulated genes	The results are almost not comparable as different time points (after intoxication with the three agents), and gene classifications have been chosen in the three animal models.
Genomic responses	Sox11	Bcl X	IL-6	
	α-prothymosin	Bcl2I11	TNF-α	
	Protein kinase C receptor	Casp6	ATF3	
	Neuropeptide Y	Gabrr2	KLF4	
	Thymosin-β-10	Hsd17b1	NR4A3	
	CD9	Arrb1	CREM	
	CD24	Scrd3	IER2	
	β - tubulin	Mapk 14	CCNL1	
	T- β -15 Vimentin	Calcr	IMPACT	
	Fatty acid binding protein	Scya2	PP1R15A	
		Camk2d	DUSP5	
		Calm	Hsp70	
		S100b	MKL1	
		Cncg	HSPA1A	
		Clc-k2I	HSPA1A	
		ClCn5	CCNK	
		Scn2b	RBPMS	
		Accn2	NFKBIZ	
		Kcnh2	TLR7	
		IL-10	TNFRSF1A	
		Cish3	IFNGR1	
		Tgfa	SLC25A3	
		CD40I	STAT3	
		Pip1	CEBPD	
		Mbp	TGIF1	
		Kcnj1	MEF2C	
		Apoe	MAPKAPK2	
		Atplb2		
	Down-regulated genes	**Down-regulated genes**	**Down-regulated genes**	
	GAS-7	Thra	FGF9	
	R-esp1	Ptger3	GRAP2	
	NVP-2	Gria2	DGKZ	
	PDK2	Adrbk1	PTPN3	
	PMCA-3	Stx6	GPT	
	Hippocalcin	SVOP	PSCD3	
	Inositol 1,4,5-triphosphate receptor	Synj1	PTCD3	
		Hsp25	TNFAIP8	
	Type II calcium/calmodulin-dependent protein Kinase-β subunit	Camk2a	AIFM1	
		Cacna1a	EXT2	
		Kcnd3	TRIM32	
		Pcp2858	ADNP	
		c-Kit	MKL1	
	GABA-A receptor-Δ subunit	Nfyc	FCGRT	
	Prodynorphin	Kras2	AKR1C14	
	Spinophilin	Nefh	ECHS1	
	Dendrin	Atpla1	SYNE	
	D-dopachrome tautomerase			
	Neural membrane protein 35			

Long-term effects on behavioral response	Learning and memory impairment, depression and anxiety	Learning and sensorimotor impairment, stress, enhanced acoustic startle, increase in overall activity. Repeated sarin exposure may disrupt normal sleeping patterns. In human, symptomatic sequelae in the higher and visual nervous system, delayed effects on psychomotor performance and memory decline occur following the sarin poisoning	Learning impairment and anxiety	Learning impairment and anxiety	Sarin induces enhanced acoustic startle, sensorimotor impairment in rat model, and symptomatic sequelae in the higher and visual nervous system, and memory decline in human

REFERENCES

[1]   Wood SJ, Tattersall JE. An improved brain slice model of nerve agent-induced seizure activity. J Appl Toxicol 2001; 21 (Suppl 1): S83-6.

[2]   Tetz LM, Rezk PE, Ratcliffe RH, Gordon RK, Steele KE, Nambiar MP. Development of a rat pilocarpine model of seizure/status epilepticus that mimics chemical warfare nerve agent exposure. Toxicol Ind Health 2006; 22: 255-66.

[3]   Turski WA, Cavalheiro EA, Schwarz M, Czuczwar SJ, Kleinrok Z, Turski L. Limbic seizures produced by pilocarpine in rats: behavioural, electroencephalographic and neuropathological study. Behav Brain Res 1983; 9: 315-35.

[4]   Turski WA, Cavalheiro EA, Bortolotto ZA, Mello LM, Schwarz M, Turski L. Seizures produced by pilocarpine in mice: a behavioral, electroencephalographic and morphological analysis. Brain Res 1984; 321: 237-53.

[5]   Turski WA, Cavalheiro EA, Coimbra C, da Penha Berzaghi M, Ikonomidou-Turski, Turski L. Only certain antiepileptic drugs prevent seizures induced by pilocarpine. Brain Res 1987; 434: 281-305.

[6]   Turski L, Ikonomidou C, Turski WA, Bortolotto ZA, Cavalheiro EA. Review: cholinergic mechanisms and epileptogenesis. The seizures induced by pilocarpine: a novel experimental model of intractable epilepsy. Synapse 1989; 3: 154-71.

[7]   Cavalheiro EA, Leite JP, Bortolotto, ZA, Turski WA, Turski L. Long-term effects of pilocarpine in rats: structural damage of the brain triggers kindling and spontaneous recurrent seizures. Epilepsia 1991; 32: 778–782.

[8]   Cavalheiro EA, Santos NF, Priel MR. The pilocarpine model of epilepsy in mice. Epilepsia 1996; 37: 1015-9.

[9]   Tang FR, Lee WL, Yang J, Sim MK, Ling EA. Expression of metabotropic glutamate receptor 1alpha in the hippocampus of rat pilocarpine model of status epilepticus. Epilepsy Res 2001; 46: 179-89.

[10]   Tang FR, Lee WL, Gao H, Chen Y, Loh YT, Chia SC, Expression of different isoforms of protein kinase C in the rat hippocampus after pilocarpine induced status epilepticus with special reference to CA1 area and the dentate gyrus. Hippocampus 2004; 14: 87-98.

[11]   Tang FR, Chia SC, Zhang S *et al.* Glutamate receptor 1 immunopositive neurons in the gliotic CA1 area of the mouse hippocampus after pilocarpine induced status epilepticus. Eur J Neurosci 2005; 21: 2361-74

[12]   Tang FR, Chia SC, Jiang FL, Ma DL, Chen PM, Tang YC, Calcium binding protein immunopositive neurons in the gliotic hippocampus of the mouse model of epilepsy with special reference to their afferents from the medial septum and nucleus of the diagonal band of Broca. Neuroscience 2006; 140: 1467-1479.

[13]   Tang FR, Chen PM, Tang YC, Tsai MC, Lee WL. Two-methyl-6-phenylethynyl-pyridine (MPEP), a metabotropic glutamate receptor 5 antagonist, with low doses of MK801 and diazepam: a novel approach for controlling status epilepticus. Neuropharmacology 2007; 53: 821-31.

[14]   Ma DL, Tang YC, Chen PM *et al.* Reorganization of CA3 area of the mouse hippocampus after pilocarpine induced temporal lobe epilepsy with special reference to the CA3-septum pathway. J Neurosci Res 2006; 83: 318-331.

[15] Ma DL, Tang YC, Tang FR. Cytoarchitectonics and afferent/efferent reorganization of the lateral entorhinal cortex in the mouse pilocarpine model of temporal lobe epilepsy. J Neurosci Res 2008; 86: 1324-1342.

[16] Zhang S, Khanna S, Tang FR. Patterns of hippocampal neuronal loss and axon reorganization of the dentate gyrus in the mouse pilocarpine model of temporal lobe epilepsy J Neurosci Res 2009; 87: 1135-1149.

[17] Liu JX, Cao X, Tang YC, Liu Y, Tang FR. CCR7, CCR8, CCR9 and CCR10 in the mouse hippocampal CA1 area and the dentate gyrus during and after pilocarpine-induced status epilepticus. J Neurochem 2007; 100: 1072-88.

[18] Liu JX, Tang YC, Liu Y, Tang FR. mGluR5-PLCβ4-PKCβ2/PKCγ pathways in hippocampal CA1 pyramidal neurons in pilocarpine model of status epilepticus in mGluR5+/+ mice. Epilepsy Res 2008; 82: 111-123.

[19] Liu JX, Tang YC, Liu Y, Tang FR. Status epilepticus alters hippocampal PKAbeta and PKAgamma expression in mice. Seizure 2010; 19: 414-20.

[20] Xu JH, Long L, Tang YC, Zhang JT, Hut HT, Tang FR. CCR3, CCR2A and macrophage inflammatory protein (MIP)-1a, monocyte chemotactic protein-1 (MCP-1) in the mouse hippocampus during and after pilocarpine-induced status epilepticus (PISE). Neuropathol Appl Neurobiol 2009; 35: 496-514.

[21] Xu JH, Long L, Tang YC, Hu HT, Tang FR. Ca(v)1.2, Ca(v)1.3, and Ca(v)2.1 in the mouse hippocampus during and after pilocarpine-induced status epilepticus. Hippocampus 2007; 17: 235-51.

[22] Xu JH, Long L, Wang J *et al.* Nuclear localization of Ca(v)2.2 and its distribution in the mouse central nervous system, and changes in the hippocampus during and after pilocarpine-induced status epilepticus. Neuropathol Appl Neurobiol 2010; 36:71-85.

[23] He DF, Ma DL, Tang YC *et al.* Morpho-physiological characteristics of dorsal subicular network in mice after pilocarpine induced status epilepticus. Brain Pathol 2010: 20: 80-95.

[24] Davies SG, Roberts PM, Stephenson PT, Thomson JE. Syntheses of the racemic jaborandi alkaloids pilocarpine, isopilocarpine and pilosinine. Tetrahedron Letters 2009; 50: 3509-3512.

[25] Wollensak J, Kewitz H. One hundred years pilocarpine in ophthalmology Klin Monatsbl Augenheilkd 1976; 169: 660-3.

[26] Smith DJ, Taubman MA, Ebersole JL, King W. Relationship between frequency of pilocarpine administration and salivary IgA level. J Dent Res 1982; 61: 1451-3.

[27] Cordner SM, Fysh RR, Gordon H, Whitaker SJ. Deaths of two hospital inpatients poisoned by pilocarpine. Br Med J 1986; 293: 1285-7.

[28] Andre MJ. Two cases of fatal poisoning with pilocarpine in normal doses. Conania Neurologica 1949; 10: 8-21.

[29] Tang FR, Chia SC, Chen PM *et al.* Metabotropic glutamate receptor 2/3 in the hippocampus of patients with mesial temporal lobe epilepsy, and of rats and mice after pilocarpine-induced status epilepticus. Epilepsy Res 2004; 59: 167-80.

[30] Tang FR. Agonists and antagonists of metabotropic glutamate receptors: anticonvulsants and antiepileptogenic agents? Current Neuropharmacology 2005; 3: 299-307.

[31] Jiang FL, Tang YC, Chia SC, Jay TM, Tang FR. Anti-convulsive effect of a selective metabotropic glutamate receptor 8 agonist (S)-3,4-dicarboxyphenylglycines (S-3,4-DCPG) in the mouse pilocarpine model of status epilepticus. Epilepsia 2007; 48: 783-92.

[32] Tang FR, Bradford HF, Ling EA. Metabotropic glutamate receptors in the control of neuronal activity and as targets for development of anti-epileptogenic drugs. Curr Med Chem 2009; 16: 2189-204.

[33] Donzanti BA, Green MD, Shores EI. Atropine sulfate and 2-pyridine aldoxime methylchloride elicit stress-induced convulsions and lethality in mice and guinea pigs. Drug Chem Toxicol 1985; 8: 431-49.

[34] Somani SM, Solana RP, Dube SN. Toxicodynamics of Nerve Agents In: Somani SM Ed., Chemical warfare agents. San Diego, California: Academic Press Inc. 1992; pp 68-108

[35] Prenant C, Crouzel C, Synthesis of [11C]-sarin. Journal of Radiolabelled Compounds and Radiopharmaceuticals 1990; 18: 645–651.

[36] Jope RS, Morrisett RA, Snead OC, Characterization of lithium potentiation of pilocarpine-induced status epilepticus in rats. Exp Neurol 1986; 91: 471-480

[37] Smolders I, Khan GM, Manil J. Ebinger G, Michotte Y. NMDA receptor-mediated pilocarpine-induced seizures: characterization in freely moving rats by microdialysis. Br J Pharmacol 1997; 121: 1171-9.

[38] Meurs A, Clinckers R, Ebinger G, Michotte Y, Smolders I. Seizure activity and changes in hippocampal extracellular glutamate, GABA, dopamine and serotonin. Epilepsy Res 2008; 78: 50-9.

[39] Ormandy GC, Jope RS, Snead OC 3rd. Anticonvulsant actions of MK-801 on the lithium-pilocarpine model of status epilepticus in rats. Exp Neurol 1989; 106: 172-80.

[40] Smolders I, Bortolotto ZA, Clarke VR *et al.* Antagonists of GLU(K5)-containing kainate receptors prevent pilocarpine-induced limbic seizures. Nat Neurosci 2002; 5: 796-804.

[41] al-Tajir G, Starr MS. Anticonvulsant effect of striatal dopamine D2 receptor stimulation: dependence on cortical circuits? Neuroscience 1991; 43: 51-7.

[42]   Houser CR, Esclapez M, Vulnerability and plasticity of the GABA system in the pilocarpine model of spontaneous recurrent seizures. Epilepsy Res 1996; 26: 207-18.

[43]   Khan GM, Smolders I, Ebinger G, Michotte Y. Anticonvulsant effect and neurotransmitter modulation of focal and systemic 2-chloroadenosine against the development of pilocarpine-induced seizures. Neuropharmacology 2000; 39: 2418-32.

[44]   Marinho MM, de Bruin VM, de Sousa FC, Aguiar LM, de Pinho RS, Viana GS. Inhibitory action of a calcium channel blocker (nimodipine) on seizures and brain damage induced by pilocarpine and lithium-pilocarpine in rats. Neurosci Lett 1997; 235: 13-6.

[45]   Shih TM, McDonough JH Jr. Neurochemical mechanisms in soman-induced seizures. J Appl Toxicol 1997; 17: 255-64.

[46]   Capacio BR, Shih TM. Anticonvulsant actions of anticholinergic drugs in soman poisoning. Epilepsia 1991; 32: 604–615.

[47]   McDonough JH Jr, Shih TM. Neuropharmacological mechanisms of nerve agent-induced seizure and neuropathology. Neurosci Biobehav Rev 1997; 21: 559–579.

[48]   Lallement G, Pernot-Marino I, Foquin-Tarricone A, Baubichon D, Piras A, Blanchet G, Carpentier P. Antiepileptic effects of NBQX against soman-induced seizures. Neuroreport 1994; 5: 425-8.

[49]   Apland JP, Aroniadou-Anderjaska V, Braga MF. Soman induces ictogenesis in the amygdala and interictal activity in the hippocampus that are blocked by a GluR5 kainate receptor antagonist *in vitro*. Neuroscience 2009; 159: 380-9.

[50]   Al-Tajir G, Starr MS. Anticonvulsant action of SCH 23390 in the striatum of the rat. European Journal of Pharmacology 1990; 191: 329–336.

[51]   Bourne JA. SCH 23390: the first selective dopamine D1-like receptor antagonist. CNS Drug Rev 2001; 7: 399-414.

[52]   Gale K. Role of GABA in the genesis of chemoconvulsant seizures. Toxicol Lett 1992; 64-65: 417–428.

[53]   Bodjarian N, Carpentier P, Baubichon D, Blanchet G, Lallement G. Involvement of non-muscarinic receptors in phosphoinositide signalling during soman-induced seizures. Eur J Pharmacol 1995; 289: 291-7.

[54]   Shih TM, McDonough JH Jr. Organophosphorus nerve agents-induced seizures and efficacy of atropine sulfate as anticonvulsant treatment. Pharmacol Biochem Behav 1999; 64: 147-53.

[55]   Harrison PK, Bueters TJ, Ijzerman AP, van Helden HP, Tattersall JE. Partial adenosine A(1) receptor agonists inhibit sarin-induced epileptiform activity in the hippocampal slice. Eur J Pharmacol 2003; 471: 97-104.

[56]   Tuovinen K. Organophosphate-induced convulsions and prevention of neuropathological damages. Toxicology 2004; 196: 31-9.

[57]   Skovira JW, McDonough JH, Shih TM. Protection against sarin-induced seizures in rats by direct brain microinjection of scopolamine, midazolam or MK-801. J Mol Neurosci 2010; 40: 56-62

[58]   Chapman S, Kadar T, Gilat E. Seizure duration following sarin exposure affects neuro-inflammatory markers in the rat brain. NeuroToxicol 2006; 27: 277-83.

[59]   Tang FR, Lee WL. Hippocampal mossy fiber reorganization in temporal lobe epilepsy. In: Tang FR, Ed. Pan brain abnormal neural network in epilepsy, Kerala, India, Research Signpost, 2009; pp. 23-40.

[60]   Tang FR, Ma DL, Lee WL. Entorhinal cortex in temporal lobe epilepsy. In: Tang FR, Ed. Pan brain abnormal neural network in epilepsy, Kerala, India, Research Signpost, 2009; pp. 121-133.

[61]   Petras JM, Soman neurotoxicity. Fundam Appl Toxicol 1981; 1: 242.

[62]   Lemercier G, Carpentier P, Sentenac-Roumanou H, Morelis P. Histological and histochemical changes in the central nervous system of the rat poisoned with an irreversible anticholinesterase compound. Acta Neuropathol (Berl.) 1983; 61: 123-129.

[63]   McLeod CG. Pathology of nerve agents: perspectives on medical management. Fundam Appl Toxicol 1985; SlO-Sl6.

[64]   Samson FE, Pazdermik TL, Cross RS *et al.* Soman reduced changes in brain regional glucose use Fundam Appl Toxicol 1984; 4: S173-S183.

[65]   Martin LJ, Doebler JA, Shih TM, Anthony A. Protective effect of diazepam pretreatment on soman-induced brain lesion formation. Brain Res 1985; 325: 287-289.

[66]   Zimmer LA, Ennis M, el-Etri M, Shipley MT. Anatomical localization and time course of Fos expression following soman-induced seizures. J Comp Neurol 1997; 378: 468-81.

[67]   McDonough JH Jr, Clark TR, Slone TW Jr *et al.* Neural lesions in the rat and their relationship to EEG delta activity following seizures induced by the nerve agent soman. NeuroToxicol 1998; 19:381-91.

[68]   Britt JO Jr, Martin JL, Okerberg CV, Dick EJ Jr. Histopathologic changes in the brain, heart, and skeletal muscle of rhesus macaques, ten days after exposure to soman (an organophosphorus nerve agent). Comp Med 2000; 50: 133-9.

[69]   Carpentier P, Foquin A, Rondouin G, Lerner-Natoli M, de Groot DM, Lallement G. Effects of atropine sulphate on seizure activity and brain damage produced by soman in guinea-pigs: ECoG correlates of neuropathology. NeuroToxicol 2000; 21: 521-40.

[70]   Kadar T, Shapira S, Cohen G, Sahar R, Alkalay D, Raveh L. Sarin-induced neuropathology in rats. Hum Exp Toxicol 1995; 14: 252-9.

[71]   Abdel-Rahman A, Shetty AK, Abou-Donia MB. Acute exposure to sarin increases blood brain barrier permeability and induces neuropathological changes in the rat brain: dose-response relationships. Neuroscience 2002; 113: 721-41.

[72]   Grauer E, Chapman S, Rabinovitz I *et al.* Single whole-body exposure to sarin vapor in rats: long-term neuronal and behavioral deficits. Toxicol Appl Pharmacol 2008; 227: 265-74.

[73]   Parent JM, Yu TW, Leibowitz RT, Geschwind DH, Sloviter RS, Lowenstein DH. Dentate granule cell neurogenesis is increased by seizures and contributes to aberrant network reorganization in the adult rat hippocampus. J Neurosci 1997; 17: 3727-38.

[74]   Covolan L, Ribeiro LT, Longo BM, Mello LE. Cell damage and neurogenesis in the dentate granule cell layer of adult rats after pilocarpine- or kainate-induced status epilepticus. Hippocampus 2000; 10: 169-80.

[75]   Scharfman HE, Goodman JH, Sollas AL. Granule-like neurons at the hilar/CA3 border after status epilepticus and their synchrony with area CA3 pyramidal cells: functional implications of seizure-induced neurogenesis. J Neurosci 2000; 20: 6144-58.

[76]   Tang FR, Loke WK. In: Tang BL. Ed. Neurogenesis, Neurodegeneration and Neuroregeneration. Kerala, India, Research Signpost. 2010: pp. 43-58.

[77]   Varodayan FP, Zhu XJ, Cui XN, Porter BE. Seizures increase cell proliferation in the dentate gyrus by shortening progenitor cell-cycle length. Epilepsia 2009; 50: 2638-47.

[78]   Jung KH, Chu K, Lee ST *et al.* Region-specific plasticity in the epileptic rat brain: a hippocampal and extrahippocampal analysis. Epilepsia 2009; 50: 537-49.

[79]   Hattiangady B, Rao MS, Shetty AK. Chronic temporal lobe epilepsyis associated with severely declined dentate neurogenesis in the adult hippocampus. Neurobiol Dis 2004; 17: 473-90.

[80]   Hattiangady B, Shetty AK. Implications of decreased hippocampal neurogenesis in chronic temporal lobe epilepsy. Epilepsia 2008; 49 (Suppl 5): 26-41.

[81]   Hattiangady B, Shetty AK. Decreased neuronal differentiation of newly generated cells underlies reduced hippocampal neurogenesis in chronic temporal lobe epilepsy. Hippocampus 2010; 20: 97-112.

[82]   Collombet JM, Four E, Bernabé D *et al.* Soman poisoning increases neural progenitor proliferation and induces long-term glial activation in mouse brain. Toxicology 2005; 208: 319-34.

[83]   Filliat P, Coubard S, Pierard C *et al.* Long-term behavioral consequences of soman poisoning in mice. NeuroToxicol 2007; 28: 508-519.

[84]   Joosen MJ, Jousma E, van den Boom TM, Kuijpers WC, Smit AB, Lucassen PJ, van Helden HP. Long-term cognitive deficits accompanied by reduced neurogenesis after soman poisoning. NeuroToxicol 2009; 30: 72-80.

[85]   Kawabuchi M, Cintra WM, Deshpande SS, Albuquerque EX. Morphological and electrophysiological study of distal motor nerve fiber degeneration and sprouting after irreversible cholinesterase inhibition. Synapse. 1991; 8: 218-28.

[86]   Becker AJ, Chen J, Zien A *et al.* Correlated stage- and subfield-associated hippocampal gene expression patterns in experimental and human temporal lobe epilepsy. Eur J Neurosci 2003; 18: 2792-802.

[87]   Elliott RC, Miles MF, Lowenstein DH. Overlapping microarray profiles of dentate gyrus gene expression during development- and epilepsy-associated neurogenesis and axon outgrowth. J Neurosci 2003; 23: 2218-27.

[88]   Dillman JF 3rd, Phillips CS, Kniffin DM, Tompkins CP, Hamilton TA, Kan RK. Gene expression profiling of rat hippocampus following exposure to the acetylcholinesterase inhibitor soman. Chem Res Toxicol 2009; 22: 633-8.

[89]   Damodaran TV, Patel AG, Greenfield ST, Dressman HK, Lin S. M, Abou-Donia MB. Gene expression profiles of the rat brain both immediately and 3 months following acute sarin exposure. Biochem Pharmacol 2006; 71: 497–520.

[90]   Damodaran TV, Greenfield ST, Patel AG, Dressman HK, Lin SK, Abou-Donia MB. Toxicogenomic studies of the rat brain at an early time point following acute sarin exposure. Neurochem Res 2006; 31: 367–381.

[91]   Leite JP, Nakamura EM, Lemos T, Masur J, Cavalheiro EA. Learning impairment in chronic epileptic rats following pilocarpine-induced status epilepticus. Braz J Med Biol Res 1990; 23: 681-3.

[92]   Bernardi RB, Barros HM. Carbamazepine enhances discriminative memory in a rat model of epilepsy. Epilepsia 2004; 45: 1443-7.

[93]   Gröticke I, Hoffmann K, Löscher W. Behavioral alterations in the pilocarpine model of temporal lobe epilepsy in mice. Exp Neurol 2007; 207: 329-49.

[94]   Zhou JL, Zhao Q, Holmes GL. Effect of levetiracetam on visual-spatial memory following status epilepticus. Epilepsy Res 2007; 73: 65-74.

[95]   Müller CJ, Gröticke I, Bankstahl M, Löscher W. Behavioral and cognitive alterations, spontaneous seizures, and neuropathology developing after a pilocarpine-induced status epilepticus in C57BL/6 mice. Exp Neurol 2009; 219: 284-97.

[96]   Sartori CR, Pelágio FC, Teixeira SA *et al.* Effects of voluntary running on spatial memory and mature brain-derived neurotrophic factor expression in mice hippocampus after status epilepticus. Behav Brain Res 2009 203: 165-72.

[97]   dos Santos NF, Arida RM, Filho EM, Priel MR, Cavalheiro EA. Epileptogenesis in immature rats following recurrent status epilepticus. Brain Res Brain Res Rev 2000; 32: 269-76.

[98]   Rutten A, van Albada M, Silveira DC *et al.* Memory impairment following status epilepticus in immature rats: time-course and environmental effects. Eur J Neurosci 2002; 16: 501-13.

[99]   Cilio MR, Sogawa Y, Cha BH, Liu X, Huang LT, Holmes GL. Long-term effects of status epilepticus in the immature brain are specific for age and model. Epilepsia 2003; 44: 518-28.

[100]   Akman C, Zhao Q, Liu X, Holmes GL. Effect of food deprivation during early development on cognition and neurogenesis in the rat. Epilepsy Behav 2004; 5: 446-54.

[101]   Kubová H, Mares P, Suchomelová L, Brozek G, Druga R, Pitkänen A. Status epilepticus in immature rats leads to behavioural and cognitive impairment and epileptogenesis. Eur J Neurosci 2004; 19: 3255-65.

[102]   Faverjon S, Silveira DC, Fu DD *et al.* Beneficial effects of enriched environment following status epilepticus in immature rats. Neurology 2002; 59: 1356-64.

[103]   Mazarati A, Siddarth P, Baldwin RA, Shin D, Caplan R, Sankar R. Depression after status epilepticus: behavioural and biochemical deficits and effects of fluoxetine. Brain 2008; 131(Pt 8): 2071-83.

[104]   Mazarati AM, Pineda E, Shin D, Tio D, Taylor AN, Sankar R. Comorbidity between epilepsy and depression: Role of hippocampal interleukin-1beta. Neurobiol Dis 2010; 37: 461-7.

[105]   Mazarati AM, Shin D, Kwon YS *et al.* Elevated plasma corticosterone level and depressive behavior in experimental temporal lobe epilepsy. Neurobiol Dis 2009; 34: 457-61.

[106]   Krishnakumar A, Nandhu MS, Paulose CS. Upregulation of 5-HT2C receptors in hippocampus of pilocarpine-induced epileptic rats: antagonism by Bacopa monnieri. Epilepsy Behav 2009; 16: 225-30.

[107]   Wolthuis OL, Vanwersch RA. Behavioral changes in the rat after low doses of cholinesterase inhibitors. Fundam Appl Toxicol 1984; 4(2 Pt 2): S195-208.

[108]   Coubard S, Béracochéa D, Collombet JM *et al.* Long-term consequences of soman poisoning in mice: part 2. Emotional behavior. Behav Brain Res 2008; 191: 95-103.

[109]   Dawson RM. Review of oximes available for treatment of nerve agent poisoning. J Appl Toxicol 1994; 14: 317–31.

[110]   Anderson DR, Harris LW, Chang FC *et al.* Antagonism of soman-induced convulsions by midazolam, diazepam and scopolamine. Drug Chem Toxicol 1997; 20: 115–31.

[111]   Shih T, McDonough JH Jr, Koplovitz I. Anticonvulsants for soman-induced seizure activity. J Biomed Sci 1999; 6: 86–96.

[112]   van Helden HP, Bueters TJ. Protective activity of adenosine receptor agonists in the treatment of organophosphate poisoning. Trends Pharmacol Sci 1999; 20: 438–41.

[113]   Landauer MR, Romano JA. Acute behavioral toxicity of the organophosphate sarin in rats. Neurobehav Toxicol Teratol 1984; 6: 239-43.

[114]   Kassa J, Koupilová M, Vachek J. Long-term effects of low-level sarin inhalation exposure on the spatial memory of rats in a T-maze. Acta Medica (Hradec Kralove). 2001; 44: 93-6.

[115]   Kassa J, Koupilová M, Vachek J. The influence of low-level sarin inhalation exposure on spatial memory in rats. Pharmacol Biochem Behav 2001; 70: 175-9.

[116]   Kassa J, Krejcová G, Vachek J. The impairment of spatial memory following low-level sarin inhalation exposure and antidotal treatment in rats. Acta Medica (Hradec Kralove). 2002; 45: 149-53.

[117]   Genovese RF, Mioduszewski RJ, Benton BJ, Pare MA, Cooksey JA. Behavioral evaluation of rats following low-level inhalation exposure to sarin. Pharmacol Biochem Behav 2009; 91: 517-25.

[118]   Yanai J, Pinkas A, Seidler FJ, Ryde IT, Van der Zee EA, Slotkin TA. Neurobehavioral teratogenicity of sarin in an avian model. Neurotoxicol Teratol. 2009; 31: 406-12.

[119]   Shih TM, Hulet SW, McDonough JH. The effects of repeated low-dose sarin exposure. Toxicol Appl Pharmacol 2006; 215: 119-34.

[120]   Murata K, Araki S, Yokoyama K, Okumura T, Ishimatsu S, Takasu N, White RF. Asymptomatic sequelae to acute sarin poisoning in the central and autonomic nervous system 6 months after the Tokyo subway attack. J Neurol 1997; 244: 601-6.

[121]   Yokoyama K, Araki S, Murata K *et al.* Chronic neurobehavioral effects of Tokyo subway sarin poisoning in relation to posttraumatic stress disorder. Arch Environ Health. 1998; 53: 249-56.

[122]   Yokoyama K, Araki S, Murata K, Nishikitani M, Okumura T, Ishimatsu Takasu N, Chronic neurobehavioral and central and autonomic nervous system effects of Tokyo subway sarin poisoning. Journal de Physiologie Paris 1998; 92: 317–323.

[123]   Nishiwaki Y, Maekawa K, Ogawa Y, Asukai N, Minami M, Omae K. Effects of sarin on the nervous system in rescue team staff members and police officers 3 years after the Tokyo subway sarin attack. Environmental Health Perspectives 2001; 109: 1169–1173.

[124] Miyaki K, Nishiwaki Y, Maekawa K *et al.* Effects of sarin on the nervous system of subway workers seven years after the Tokyo subway sarin attack. J Occup Health 2005; 47: 299–304.

[125] Sirkka U, Nieminen SA, Ylitalo P. Neurobehavioral toxicity with low doses of sarin and soman. Methods Find Exp Clin Pharmacol. 1990; 12: 245-50.

[126] Nieminen SA, Lecklin A, Heikkinen O, Ylitalo P. Acute behavioural effects of the organophosphates sarin and soman in rats. Pharmacol Toxicol 1990; 67: 36-40.

[127] Scremin OU, Shih TM, Huynh L, Roch M, Booth R, Jenden DJ. Delayed neurologic and behavioral effects of subtoxic doses of cholinesterase inhibitors. J Pharmacol Exp Ther 2003; 304: 1111-9.

[128] Abou-Donia MB, Dechkovskaia AM, Goldstein LB, Bullman SL, Khan WA. Sensorimotor deficit and cholinergic changes following coexposure with pyridostigmine bromide and sarin in rats. Toxicol Sci 2002; 66: 148-58.

[129] Yokoyama K, Araki S, Murata K *et al.* A preliminary study on delayed vestibulo-cerebellr effects of Tokyo subway sarin poisoning in relation to gender difference: frequency analysis of postural sway. J Occup Environ Med 1998; 40: 17–21.

[130] Tochigi M, Umekage T, Otani T *et al.* Serum cholesterol, uric acid and cholinesterase in victims of the Tokyo subway sarin poisoning: a relation with post-traumatic stress disorder. Neurosci Res 2002; 44: 267-72.

[131] Ohtani T, Iwanami A, Kasai K *et al.* Post-traumatic stress disorder symptoms in victims of Tokyo subway attack: a 5-year follow-up study. Psychiatry Clin Neurosci 2004; 58: 624-9.

[132] Tang FR, Lee WL. Expression of the group II and III metabotropic glutamate receptors in the hippocampus of patients with mesial temporal lobe epilepsy. J Neurocytol 2001; 30: 135-141.

[133] Tang FR, Lee WL, Yeo TT. Expression of the group I metabotropic glutamate receptor in the hippocampus of patients with mesial temporal lobe epilepsy. J Neurocytol 2001; 30: 403-411.

[134] Scremin OU, Shih TM, Li MG, Jenden DJ. Mapping of cerebral metabolic activation in three models of cholinergic convulsions. Brain Res Bull 1998; 45: 167-74.

Index

A

Aetiology 51-55, 69
Animal models 12-14; 68-76, 80-83
Axonal and dendritic architectonic changes 81-82, 94
AY-9944 75-76

B

Behavioral response 42-44, 96-97, 101
Pathology 50-51, 80-83, 92-93, 98-99

C

Carbon monoxide 13
Chemistry 89-90
Cyanide 13, 22-23

D

Diagnosis 33-34
Dopaminergic system 53

G

GABAergic system: 52-53
Gamma-Hydroxy-Butyrate 72-74
Gamma-Butyrolactone 72-74
General principles of seizures and epileptogenesis 3-4, 98
Genomic responses 94-96, 100
Glutamatergic system 51-52

K

Kainic acid 80-85

L

Life support measures 20-21

M

Mechanisms of chemically induced seizures and epileptogenesis 10-12, 30, 40-42, 68, 83-84, 98
Methylazoxymethanol acetate (MAM)-AY 76
Muscarinic syndrome 34

N

Neuroanatomy and electrophysiology 4-7
Neurogenesis 42-43, 93-94, 99
Neurotoxicology 8-10